# RUBY ROSE

# Macro Hacks For Men

*The Blueprint to Building Your Best Body*

*Dedication*

*To every man who has ever felt stuck, confused, or defeated on their fitness journey—this book is for you.*

*To the relentless dreamers who dare to believe in their best selves, and to the quiet achievers who prove every day that change is possible with consistency and courage.*

*And to my family, friends, and mentors—thank you for your unwavering support and belief in this vision. Your strength and encouragement inspire me to keep building, learning, and sharing.*

# Contents

# Introduction

Imagine a life where you feel unstoppable—where your body is not only strong but functions like a finely tuned machine. Whether you're an athlete aiming for peak performance, someone on a fat loss journey, or simply looking to embrace a healthier lifestyle, your success starts here. Macro Hacks: The Blueprint to Building Your Best Body isn't just another fitness guide; it's your ultimate toolkit for achieving transformative results through the power of macronutrient nutrition.

This book is built on a simple truth: knowledge is power. In the world of fitness and nutrition, macronutrients—carbohydrates, proteins, and fats—are the currency of success. But not all macros are created equal, and understanding how to tailor them to your unique goals is the game-changer you've been looking for. With clear explanations, practical strategies, and cutting-edge science, Macro Hacks empowers you to take charge of your diet, optimize your energy, and unlock your body's full potential.

Gone are the days of fad diets and guesswork. This is a proven, science-backed approach that demystifies calories, reveals the secrets of sustainable weight management, and shows you how to build muscle, burn fat, and improve overall health. From crafting your unique macro profile to mastering advanced techniques for fine-tuning your intake, this book is your step-by-step guide to long-term success.

You'll find actionable advice on overcoming common nutrition challenges, creating personalized meal plans, and building habits that stick. Whether it's fueling your workouts with the right carbs, harnessing the power of protein for muscle growth, or understanding the essential role of healthy fats, this book meets you where you are and equips you with everything you need to succeed.

Are you ready to stop dieting and start thriving? With Macro Hacks For Men as your blueprint, the best version of you is just a page away.

# The Macro Blueprint

## Why Macros Matter

### 1.1 Understanding the Basics: What Are Macros?

Have you ever heard fitness enthusiasts obsess over their "macros" and wondered what the fuss was about? Macros, short for macronutrients, are the building blocks of the food we eat. They consist of three primary categories: carbohydrates, proteins, and fats. Each serves a distinct purpose in fueling your body and supporting your health. Understanding macros is like decoding the language of nutrition—it's the first step toward taking control of your diet and fitness journey.

Carbohydrates, often misunderstood as the villain of many trendy diets, are your body's primary source of energy. Found in foods like bread, rice, fruits, and vegetables, they're broken down into glucose to power everything from your workouts to your daily tasks. Proteins, the heroes of muscle recovery and repair, are composed of amino acids. They are found in meat, fish, eggs, and plant-based sources like beans and lentils. Lastly, fats, often unfairly demonized, are crucial for hormone production, brain function, and energy storage. Healthy fats are abundant in nuts, seeds, avocados, and fatty fish.

Each gram of carbs and protein provides four calories, while fats pack a punch at nine calories per gram. This calorie difference is important because it helps you plan a balanced diet tailored to your goals. Whether you're trying to lose fat, build muscle, or maintain your weight, knowing the role of each macro can help you make smarter choices.

But here's the real secret: not all macros are created equal. A sugary donut and a bowl of oatmeal both contain carbs, but their impact on your energy levels and body composition is worlds apart. By understanding the quality of macros and how they fit into your lifestyle, you can set the foundation for achieving your best body. Knowledge is power, and in this case, it's also the key to unlocking a fitter, healthier you.

## 1.2 Nutrition vs. Results: The Macro-Fitness Connection

You've been hitting the gym religiously, but the results are slower than you'd hoped. What gives? The answer often lies in your diet. While workouts are vital for building strength and endurance, your nutrition is the driving force behind visible results. Macros are the missing puzzle piece that bridges the gap between effort and outcome.

When you consume the right balance of macros, your body operates like a well-oiled machine. Carbs supply the energy you need to crush your workouts, proteins repair the micro-tears in your muscles, and fats keep your hormones in check, ensuring your metabolism stays efficient. Neglecting any of these can throw your progress off course. For instance, cutting carbs too drastically might leave you feeling sluggish, while a lack of protein can hinder muscle recovery, leading to plateaus.

Think of macros as the architects of your physique. If you want to build muscle, you'll need a protein-rich diet to provide the raw materials for growth. Pair this with sufficient carbs for energy and fats for recovery, and you've got a recipe for success. On the flip side, if fat loss is your goal, a calorie deficit is key, but the macro breakdown ensures you lose fat—not muscle. By prioritizing protein and balancing your carbs and fats, you can sculpt a leaner, more defined body.

Scientific studies back this up. A meta-analysis published in the Journal of Sports Nutrition found that individuals who followed macro-based eating plans had better body composition results than those who simply counted calories. Why? Because macros determine how your body uses those calories. A protein-rich meal triggers muscle synthesis, while a carb-heavy snack replenishes glycogen stores. Understanding these nuances helps you fuel your body for the outcomes you desire.

So, if you've ever wondered why your workouts alone aren't cutting it, it's time to take a closer look at your plate. Dialing in your macros isn't just about eating; it's about eating with purpose.

## 1.3 The Science of Body Composition: Fat Loss and Muscle Gain

What if you could lose fat and gain muscle simultaneously? It might sound like magic, but it's actually the science of body composition—and macros play a starring role. Your body is constantly in a state of building and breaking down tissue, and your macro intake determines which process dominates.

Protein is the cornerstone of muscle growth. When you strength train, you create micro-tears in your muscle fibers. Protein repairs these tears, making your muscles stronger and larger. Consuming enough protein is non-negotiable if you're serious about gains. Aim for around 0.8 to 1 gram of protein per pound of body weight daily, and watch your muscles thrive.

Carbs are your muscles' best friend, despite what low-crab diets might claim. They replenish glycogen stores depleted during workouts, giving you the energy to train harder and recover faster. Without enough carbs, your body might turn to breaking down muscle tissue for energy—a process you definitely want to avoid.

Fats, often misunderstood, are the unsung heroes of fat loss. Hormones like testosterone and growth hormone, which are critical for muscle gain and fat loss, are produced with the help of dietary fats. Including healthy fats in your diet supports these processes, ensuring your body is primed for success.

The key to achieving your desired body composition lies in creating the right balance. If fat loss is your priority, you'll need a calorie deficit—burning more energy than you consume. But here's the twist: cutting calories recklessly can backfire by causing muscle loss. By maintaining a higher protein intake and balancing carbs and fats, you signal your body to hold onto lean muscle while shedding fat.

On the flip side, if muscle gain is your goal, a calorie surplus is necessary, but it must be controlled. Excessive overeating can lead to fat gain, negating your hard work in the gym. A slight surplus, paired with the right macro breakdown, ensures your gains are lean and sustainable.

Macros are the ultimate tool for reshaping your body. They're not just numbers on a nutrition label—they're the blueprint for unlocking your best physique.

# Understanding the Big Picture

## 2.1 The Three Macronutrients: Protein, Carbs, and Fats

Macronutrients, or macros, are the cornerstone of your diet, dictating how your body functions, performs, and transforms. To harness their power, you need to understand each one individually: protein, carbohydrates, and fats.

These three macros work synergistically to fuel your body, repair tissues, and regulate processes vital for health and fitness.

Protein is often hailed as the building block of life—and for good reason. Made up of amino acids, protein is essential for repairing and building tissues, especially muscle. Think of it as the construction crew for your body, fixing wear and tear and helping you grow stronger. Sources include lean meats, fish, eggs, dairy, and plant-based options like tofu, lentils, and quinoa. Consuming adequate protein is vital for anyone aiming to build muscle, recover from workouts, or maintain overall health.

Carbohydrates, on the other hand, are your body's primary energy source. Whether you're running a marathon or tackling a busy workday, carbs provide the fuel you need. They break down into glucose, which your cells use for energy. But not all carbs are created equal. Simple carbs, like sugar, offer a quick burst of energy, while complex carbs, such as whole grains and vegetables, provide sustained fuel. The key is choosing the right type and quantity to match your activity level and goals.

Fats, often misunderstood, are critical for long-term health and peak performance. Healthy fats support hormone production, brain function, and energy storage. They're particularly important for athletes and individuals focusing on fat loss or muscle gain. Found in avocados, nuts, seeds, and fatty fish, fats also enhance the absorption of fat-soluble vitamins like A, D, E, and K.

Understanding the unique role of each macronutrient is the first step toward optimizing your diet. Together, they form the nutritional trifecta that powers your workouts, supports recovery, and helps you achieve your fitness goals. By treating macros as tools rather than obstacles, you can take a significant step toward building your best body.

## 2.2 Balancing Act: The Importance of Balanced Macro Intake

Imagine trying to build a house with too many bricks and not enough mortar. That's what happens when your macro intake is unbalanced. Each macronutrient has a specific role, and striking the right balance ensures they work in harmony to support your goals, whether it's fat loss, muscle gain, or overall health.

A balanced macro diet doesn't mean eating equal amounts of protein, carbs, and fats; it means adjusting your intake based on your unique needs, activity level, and goals. For instance, an athlete training for endurance will require more carbohydrates to fuel their workouts, while someone focused on fat loss might prioritize protein to preserve lean muscle.

But why is balance so crucial? Overemphasizing one macro at the expense of others can lead to issues. Too many carbs without enough protein might leave you feeling sluggish and prone to fat gain. Excessive protein without enough carbs can compromise energy levels, making it hard to perform well in workouts. Neglecting fats can disrupt hormone production, leading to fatigue and impaired recovery.

Scientific studies support the importance of balance. Research in the American Journal of Clinical Nutrition found that diets with a balanced macro ratio led to better weight management and improved body composition compared to extreme low-carb or low-fat diets. Balance also supports long-term sustainability. A diet overly skewed toward one macro might yield short-term results but often feels restrictive, leading to burnout.

Achieving balance doesn't require perfection—it requires awareness. Start by tracking your macros and experimenting with ratios to find what works best for you. Tools like macro calculators can provide a personalized starting point, but listening to your body is equally important. Energy levels, workout performance, and overall mood are great indicators of whether your macro balance is on point.

Ultimately, balance is about creating a diet that fuels your goals without sacrificing your well-being. By honoring the unique role of each macronutrient and finding harmony among them, you can build a sustainable lifestyle that delivers results.

## 2.3 Macro Myths Debunked: Common Misconceptions About Macros

The world of macros is rife with myths, often fueled by misinformation and fad diets. These misconceptions can derail your progress and leave you frustrated. Let's bust some of the most common macro myths so you can focus on what truly works.

**Myth 1: Carbs Make You Fat**

One of the most persistent myths is that carbohydrates are the enemy. The truth? Carbs don't inherently cause fat gain—excess calories do. Carbs are your body's primary energy source, and when consumed in the right quantities, they fuel workouts and recovery. The problem arises when people overeat simple carbs like sugary snacks while neglecting complex carbs like whole grains and vegetables.

**Myth 2: High Protein Damages Your Kidneys**

Protein often gets a bad rap for supposedly harming kidney function. However, this myth is largely unfounded for healthy individuals. Research has shown that high-protein diets are safe for those without preexisting kidney conditions. In fact, athletes and active individuals require more protein to support muscle repair and growth.

**Myth 3: Fats Should Be Avoided**

Fats have long been demonized, especially during the low-fat diet craze of the 1990s. While it's true that trans fats and excessive saturated fats can harm your health, healthy fats are essential. They support hormone production, improve brain function, and even aid in fat loss by keeping you satiated. Including sources like avocados, nuts, and olive oil in your diet can enhance your overall health.

**Myth 4: All Macros Are Created Equal**

A calorie is a calorie, right? Not quite. The quality of your macros matters. For example, 100 calories from processed junk food won't provide the same nutritional benefits as 100 calories from whole foods. Choosing nutrient-dense sources of protein, carbs, and fats ensures your body gets the vitamins, minerals, and fiber it needs to function optimally.

Debunking these myths is key to understanding how macros truly work. By separating fact from fiction, you can approach your diet with confidence and clarity, avoiding the pitfalls of misinformation. When it comes to macros, knowledge isn't just power—it's the secret to lasting results.

# Your Body, Your Goals

## 3.1 Defining Your Goal: Setting Clear Fitness Objectives

Before diving into the specifics of macro tracking, it's crucial to define what you're working toward. Without a clear goal, it's like embarking on a journey without a destination—you'll waste time, energy, and motivation. Whether you want to lose fat, gain muscle, or simply maintain a healthy lifestyle, defining your objective is the first step to success.

Start by asking yourself, "What do I really want?" Be specific. Saying, "I want to get fit" is too vague. Instead, aim for something measurable like, "I want to lose 10 pounds in three months," or, "I want to build 5 pounds of muscle in six months." Clear goals provide direction and help you track progress effectively.

Next, determine your why. Why is this goal important to you? Maybe you want to improve your energy levels, feel confident in your body, or set a positive example for your family. Your why is your anchor, keeping you focused and committed, especially when challenges arise.

Once your goal is defined, break it down into smaller milestones. For instance, if your ultimate aim is to lose 20 pounds, set mini-goals of 5 pounds every month. These smaller wins keep you motivated and prevent you from feeling overwhelmed.

It's also important to ensure your goals are realistic and aligned with your lifestyle. Setting overly ambitious goals, like losing 30 pounds in a month, can lead to frustration and burnout. Remember, fitness is a marathon, not a sprint. Sustainable progress always beats quick fixes.

Finally, write down your goal and revisit it often. Studies show that people who document their objectives are significantly more likely to achieve them. Pair this with a plan for accountability, such as sharing your goal with a friend or using a fitness app to track progress.

Defining your goal is about creating a clear roadmap. With the destination in mind, you're ready to align your nutrition and macros to take you there.

## 3.2 Tailoring Nutrition to Goals: Adjusting Macros for Success

Once you've defined your goal, the next step is to tailor your macro intake to match. Your body has unique needs depending on whether you're aiming for fat loss, muscle gain, or maintenance. Think of your macros as the dials on a control panel, each one adjustable to achieve your specific fitness objective.

If fat loss is your goal, you'll need to create a calorie deficit—burning more calories than you consume. However, it's not just about eating less; it's about eating strategically. Protein becomes your best friend in a fat-loss phase, as it helps preserve lean muscle while shedding fat. Aim for 0.8–1 gram of protein per pound of body weight daily. Carbs and fats should be balanced to provide energy and hormonal support, but they'll need to be slightly reduced to achieve the deficit.

For muscle gain, the opposite is true—you'll need a calorie surplus. But this doesn't mean gorging on junk food. Instead, prioritize lean proteins, complex carbs, and healthy fats to support lean muscle growth without excessive fat gain. A general rule is to consume 10–15% more calories than your maintenance level, ensuring your body has the fuel it needs for growth.

If you're maintaining your weight, focus on a balanced macro intake that matches your activity level. This is often referred to as your maintenance phase, where your calories in match your calories out. Even in maintenance, you can tweak your macros slightly to emphasize energy, recovery, or performance.

Tailoring macros also involves considering your lifestyle and preferences. If you're highly active, you might need more carbs for energy. If you're sedentary, a higher protein and fat ratio might work better. Flexibility is key—there's no one-size-fits-all approach.

Tracking your progress is crucial. Use tools like a food diary or apps to monitor your intake and adjust as needed. If your progress stalls, tweak your macros by shifting calories between carbs, fats, or proteins to reignite results.

By tailoring your nutrition to your specific goals, you're not just eating; you're eating with purpose. This alignment between diet and objective is the key to long-term success.

## 3.3 The Long-Term Vision: Making Macro Tracking a Lifestyle

Fitness is not a short-term project; it's a lifelong journey. While macro tracking might seem tedious at first, it's a skill that can transform your relationship with food and health. When approached with the right mindset, it becomes a sustainable lifestyle—not a temporary diet.

The first step toward making macro tracking a lifestyle is to focus on education. Learn to recognize portion sizes, understand food labels, and identify the macro composition of common foods. Over time, you'll develop an intuitive sense of how to balance your meals without needing to log every bite.

Next, prioritize flexibility over perfection. Life happens—birthdays, holidays, and busy schedules are inevitable. Instead of stressing over occasional slip-ups, focus on consistency. Tracking 80–90% of the time is often enough to achieve and maintain your goals. Allow yourself the freedom to enjoy treats occasionally without guilt, as this makes the lifestyle sustainable.

Another important aspect is periodically reassessing your goals and macros. As your body changes, so will your needs. For instance, if you've reached your fat loss goal and now want to focus on muscle gain, your macros will need to shift. Regularly checking in with your progress ensures you stay aligned with your objectives.

Technology can also make macro tracking easier. Apps and devices can simplify the process, helping you log meals, calculate macros, and track progress effortlessly. These tools act as a guide until you're comfortable managing your intake intuitively.

Lastly, embrace the mindset that macro tracking is not about restriction but empowerment. It's a tool that gives you control over your nutrition, allowing you to fuel your body effectively and enjoy the foods you love. By making it part of your lifestyle, you can achieve your goals while building habits that support long-term health.

Macro tracking is not a sprint but a marathon. By adopting it as a lifestyle, you're setting yourself up for lasting success, creating a healthier, stronger, and more confident version of yourself.

# Your Unique Macro Profile

## Finding Your Baseline

### 1.1 Calculating Your TDEE: Estimating Your Maintenance Calories

To achieve any fitness goal—be it weight loss, muscle gain, or maintenance—you must understand how many calories your body burns daily. This figure, known as your Total Daily Energy Expenditure (TDEE), represents the energy your body requires for all activities, from breathing to physical exercise. Calculating your TDEE is the first step in designing a macro plan tailored specifically to you.

Your TDEE calculation starts with your Basal Metabolic Rate (BMR), which measures the calories your body burns at rest. The Mifflin-St Jeor Equation is a reliable method for determining BMR. For men, the formula is . For women, it's . Once you calculate your BMR, you multiply it by an activity factor based on your lifestyle, ranging from 1.2 for a sedentary person to 1.725 for someone very active.

For example, let's calculate TDEE for a moderately active woman weighing 65 kg (143 lbs), standing 165 cm (5'5"), and aged 30. Her BMR would be . Multiplying her BMR by her activity factor (1.55 for moderate activity) gives a TDEE of calories per day. This is the number of calories she needs to maintain her current weight.

Once you've determined your TDEE, track your current caloric intake for a week. Compare your average daily intake with your TDEE. Are you eating more, less, or about the same? This simple exercise provides a clear picture of your current habits and sets the stage for meaningful adjustments. Understanding your TDEE is an essential first step in optimizing your nutrition and achieving your fitness goals.

## 1.2 Understanding Your Starting Point: Laying the Groundwork for Success

Before making changes to your diet or lifestyle, it's essential to establish your starting point. This involves assessing your current habits, caloric intake, and macronutrient distribution. Think of this step as creating a map of your current location before planning a journey. Without a clear understanding of where you are, setting and achieving realistic goals becomes much harder.

To identify your starting point, spend a week tracking everything you consume. Use a notebook or a tracking app to log your meals, snacks, and drinks, including portion sizes and hidden calories like condiments or cooking oils. Be honest and precise—this exercise is about observing your habits, not changing them. The goal is to uncover patterns in your diet and learn how they compare to your TDEE.

As you analyze your food logs, pay attention to your macronutrient ratios. How much protein, carbohydrates, and fat are you eating daily? Are your meals balanced, or are you over-relying on certain food groups? Tracking also helps you spot behaviors like overeating during stressful moments or skipping meals when you're busy. These insights are invaluable for creating a sustainable plan tailored to your lifestyle.

Establishing your starting point isn't just about gathering data; it's about setting a solid foundation for success. By understanding your current habits and caloric needs, you position yourself to make informed, targeted changes. This clarity helps you avoid the frustration of trial and error and keeps you focused on strategies that work for your body and goals.

## 1.3 The Foundation for Success: Why Starting Data Matters

Every successful fitness plan begins with accurate starting data. Without it, even the most disciplined efforts can fall short. Imagine trying to build a house without measuring the foundation—you might end up with a structure that looks good at first but eventually collapses. The same principle applies to your fitness journey.

Accurate data provides a clear picture of where you stand and serves as the foundation for all future decisions. For example, overestimating your caloric needs by just 200 calories daily could lead to weight gain over time, while underestimating them might leave you feeling fatigued and frustrated. Starting with precise numbers allows you to avoid these pitfalls and create a plan that works specifically for you.

Tracking your food intake and calculating your TDEE might seem tedious at first, but the payoff is worth it. These steps give you the tools to identify small, actionable changes that lead to significant results over time. Instead of guessing or relying on generic advice, you're making decisions based on what your body actually needs.

Think of this process as your compass. Accurate data ensures you're always moving in the right direction, even when challenges arise. It's not about perfection; it's about consistency and building a sustainable lifestyle. With this foundation in place, you're ready to tailor your macro profile and create a blueprint for achieving your best body. Let's keep building from here.

# Setting Your Macro Ratios

## 2.1 Macro Basics by Goal: Share Basic Ratios for Different Goals

Understanding macronutrient ratios is key to creating a diet tailored to your goals. Macronutrients—protein, carbohydrates, and fats—are the building blocks of your nutrition. The ratio you consume these in determines how your body responds, whether you're aiming to lose weight, build muscle, or maintain your current physique.

For weight loss, the priority is to create a calorie deficit while preserving lean muscle mass. A common starting ratio for fat loss is 40% protein, 40% carbohydrates, and 20% fats. The higher protein intake helps maintain muscle while the lower fat percentage prioritizes caloric efficiency. Carbohydrates remain moderate to fuel workouts and daily activities.

If building muscle is your goal, the focus shifts to creating a calorie surplus to support growth. In this case, a 30% protein, 50% carbohydrates, and 20% fats ratio often works well. The increased carbohydrates supply energy for intense training, while moderate protein supports muscle repair and growth. Fats are kept at a baseline level to maintain hormonal balance.

For maintenance, the goal is balancing energy intake with expenditure. A typical maintenance ratio is 30% protein, 40% carbohydrates, and 30% fats, allowing for flexibility while supporting overall health and performance. This balance is ideal for sustaining muscle, energy, and well-being.

Keep in mind, these ratios are just starting points. Individual needs vary based on factors like metabolism, lifestyle, and genetics. By understanding the role each macronutrient plays in your diet, you can tailor your ratios to align with your specific fitness goals. Setting these macros is the next step in building a plan that works for your body.

## 2.2 Adjusting for Activity Levels: Align Ratios with Physical Activity

Your activity level plays a significant role in determining how your macronutrient ratios should be adjusted. The more active you are, the more energy (and specific nutrients) your body requires. Customizing your macro ratios to reflect your activity level ensures optimal performance and recovery.

For those with a sedentary lifestyle, carbohydrates can be kept relatively low since they aren't burned as readily. A 40% protein, 30% carbohydrates, and 30% fats ratio often works well. Protein remains a priority to maintain muscle, while fats provide long-lasting energy for low activity levels.

If you engage in light activity, such as walking or yoga a few times a week, carbohydrates should be slightly higher to fuel these efforts. A 35% protein, 40% carbohydrates, and 25% fats ratio is a good starting point. This balance supports moderate energy needs without overloading on unnecessary calories.

For highly active individuals or those performing intense strength training, carbohydrates become essential. A ratio of 30% protein, 50% carbohydrates, and 20% fats ensures your muscles have enough glycogen stores to power through workouts and recover effectively.

Remember that these ratios are flexible. On particularly active days, you might increase carbohydrates slightly, while on rest days, you can reduce them to avoid excess calorie consumption. Tracking how your body responds to these adjustments will help you find the sweet spot that supports your performance and goals.

## 2.3 Learning Through Trial and Error: Refine Macros Based on Progress

Setting your initial macronutrient ratios is an important step, but the real magic happens as you refine these numbers through trial and error. Your body is unique, and what works for someone else may not work for you. Adjustments based on your progress are key to long-term success.

After setting your starting ratios, stick with them for at least two to three weeks. During this time, track your calorie intake, weight, energy levels, and performance. If your goal is fat loss, you should notice gradual changes in weight and body composition. For muscle gain, you should see an increase in weight paired with strength improvements. Maintenance should result in relatively stable weight and energy.

If you aren't seeing the desired results, it's time to tweak your ratios. For example, if fat loss has stalled, consider reducing carbohydrates slightly and increasing protein. If muscle gain isn't progressing, a small increase in carbohydrates or overall calories may be needed. The key is making small, incremental changes—too drastic of an adjustment can backfire.

Trial and error also involves listening to your body. If you feel sluggish during workouts, you might not be eating enough carbohydrates. If you're constantly hungry, adding more protein or fiber can help you feel fuller. Pay attention to how your body responds to adjustments and refine your approach accordingly.

Refining your macros is an ongoing process. As your body changes or your goals shift, your ratios may need further adjustment. Approach this process with patience and curiosity, using each tweak as an opportunity to learn what works best for you. With time, you'll develop a system that fits your lifestyle and delivers consistent results.

# Personalizing Your Approach

## 3.1 Considering Body Type: Tailor Macros to Different Body Types

When it comes to nutrition, one size doesn't fit all. Your body type—whether ectomorph, mesomorph, or endomorph—plays a significant role in how your body processes and responds to macronutrients. By tailoring your macro ratios to your body type, you can create a plan that maximizes results.

Ectomorphs are naturally lean with fast metabolisms. These individuals often struggle to gain weight or muscle mass. To support muscle growth, ectomorphs benefit from higher carbohydrates to fuel their energy demands. A good starting ratio might be 25% protein, 55% carbohydrates, and 20% fats. This ensures plenty of energy for workouts and recovery while maintaining a moderate protein intake for muscle repair.

Mesomorphs have a more athletic build and tend to respond well to exercise. They can gain muscle and lose fat relatively easily, making them well-suited for a balanced macro approach. A starting ratio of 30% protein, 40% carbohydrates, and 30% fats works well for mesomorphs, offering flexibility while supporting their body composition goals.

Endomorphs have a tendency to store fat more easily and often have a slower metabolism. To optimize fat loss or maintain weight, endomorphs typically benefit from a lower carbohydrate intake. A ratio of 35% protein, 25% carbohydrates, and 40% fats can help manage insulin levels and encourage fat burning while providing adequate energy from fats and protein.

Your body type is a helpful guideline, but it's not a rule. Many people have characteristics of multiple body types, so your initial ratios might require adjustment based on how your body responds. By starting with your body type as a framework, you can better understand what works for you and refine your approach over time.

## 3.2 Listening to Your Body: Recognize and Respond to Macro Imbalances

Your body is constantly providing feedback about how it's responding to your diet. Learning to listen to this feedback is crucial for recognizing macro imbalances and making adjustments to optimize your results.

One of the first signs of an imbalance is low energy. If you feel sluggish, especially during workouts, it may indicate you're not eating enough carbohydrates. Carbs are your body's primary energy source, and insufficient intake can leave you feeling drained. Adjusting your ratio to include more carbohydrates may improve your energy and performance.

On the other hand, frequent hunger might suggest your protein intake is too low. Protein is the most satiating macronutrient, and increasing it can help you feel fuller for longer. If your meals leave you unsatisfied or you find yourself snacking frequently, consider shifting your macro ratios to prioritize protein.

Another common sign of imbalance is weight stagnation. For example, if you're trying to lose fat but your weight isn't changing, you may be consuming too many calories or not enough protein. Conversely, if you're aiming to build muscle but not gaining weight, you might need to increase your carbohydrates or overall caloric intake.

Lastly, pay attention to digestion. Issues like bloating or discomfort could indicate an intolerance to certain foods or an imbalance in your fat or fiber intake. Adjusting your macros or food choices can often alleviate these symptoms.

Listening to your body is an ongoing process. By tuning into its signals and making thoughtful adjustments, you can create a macro plan that supports your goals while keeping you feeling your best.

## 3.3 Building a Sustainable Plan: Customize Plans to Personal Preferences

A great macro plan isn't just effective—it's also sustainable. The best plan is one you can stick to long-term without feeling restricted or overwhelmed. Customizing your macro approach to fit your preferences, lifestyle, and goals ensures it becomes a seamless part of your routine.

Start by considering your food preferences. If you enjoy carbs like pasta and bread, don't force yourself into a low-carb diet. Instead, allocate a higher percentage of your macros to carbohydrates while still staying within your caloric needs. Similarly, if you prefer richer, fatty foods like avocado or nuts, allow for a higher fat intake by reducing carbs or protein slightly.

Next, think about your schedule. If you're always on the go, focus on meals and snacks that are easy to prepare and pack. High-protein bars, pre-cooked chicken, and meal prep can help you stay on track without sacrificing convenience. For those with more time, experimenting with recipes that fit your macros can keep your meals exciting and enjoyable.

Flexibility is another key factor. Life is unpredictable, and your diet should be adaptable. For example, if you have a busy week, prioritize simple, easy-to-track meals. On weekends or special occasions, allow for indulgences and adjust your macros accordingly. The goal is to make your plan work for you—not the other way around.

Finally, remember that sustainability requires balance. Your plan should support your goals while allowing room for enjoyment. Whether it's a weekly treat or a favorite meal, including foods you love helps prevent burnout and makes the process more enjoyable.

Building a sustainable plan is about creating a lifestyle, not a temporary fix. By aligning your macros with your preferences and priorities, you set yourself up for long-term success and a healthier, happier you.

# Demystifying Calories and Energy Balance

## The Energy Equation

### 1.1 Understanding Caloric Balance: Simplify Calories In vs. Calories Out

Imagine you're standing at the crossroads of your fitness journey, overwhelmed by countless diets and trends, unsure which path will lead to success. The truth is, behind every fitness goal lies one fundamental principle: caloric balance. Mastering this concept is the key to unlocking results, whether you want to lose weight, gain muscle, or maintain your progress.

At its core, caloric balance revolves around the relationship between the energy you consume and the energy your body expends. Calories consumed through food and drink fuel everything from essential bodily functions to physical activity. On the flip side, calories burned include the energy your body uses at rest, called your Basal Metabolic Rate (BMR), and the calories spent on activities ranging from walking to intense exercise. Like a financial ledger, a surplus of calories leads to weight gain, while a deficit prompts fat loss. If the numbers even out, your weight stays the same.

Understanding caloric balance doesn't mean deprivation or extremes; it means taking control. A caloric deficit, achieved by consuming fewer calories than you burn, encourages fat loss. Meanwhile, a caloric surplus, created by eating slightly more than you expend, provides the fuel needed for muscle growth. When the balance is maintained, you stabilize your weight while optimizing energy for daily life.

The first step to applying this knowledge is becoming aware of your current intake and activity levels. Tracking your food intake and understanding your body's energy needs helps demystify why your current habits lead to specific outcomes. With these insights, you can adjust your diet and activity to align with your goals. Far from a restrictive approach, mastering caloric balance empowers you to make informed decisions, granting you the flexibility to enjoy life without sabotaging your progress.

## 1.2 Calories vs. Macros: Explain Their Relationship in Nutrition

When it comes to nutrition, calories and macronutrients often seem like competing priorities, but in reality, they are deeply interconnected. Calories measure the energy your body uses and stores, while macronutrients—protein, carbohydrates, and fats—determine how that energy is utilized. Understanding this relationship can transform how you approach your diet.

Calories are the universal currency of energy, but where those calories come from significantly affects your results. For instance, 300 calories of processed snacks fuel your body differently than 300 calories of nutrient-rich food. This difference arises from the unique roles macronutrients play in supporting your goals. Protein repairs and builds muscle, carbohydrates provide the energy needed for daily activities and workouts, and fats support vital functions like hormone regulation and brain health. The balance of these macronutrients dictates not just your caloric intake but how effectively your body performs.

To optimize your fitness journey, aligning your caloric intake with the right macronutrient ratios is crucial. If fat loss is your goal, prioritizing protein helps preserve muscle while reducing overall calorie intake. For muscle growth, a slight increase in carbohydrates and protein supports recovery and energy demands. Understanding that macros aren't separate from calories but instead define how calories work within your body adds a new layer of precision to your approach.

By focusing on nutrient-dense sources, you ensure your body receives the quality fuel it needs. This balance not only enhances physical results but also boosts your overall health. The synergy between calories and macros becomes your blueprint for building the best version of yourself, a plan tailored to your unique goals and lifestyle.

## 1.3 Why Energy Matters: Show How Energy Impacts Fitness Results

Energy is the unseen force driving your fitness results, influencing everything from how you power through workouts to how you recover afterward. Many people struggle to see progress, not because they lack effort, but because they misunderstand how energy works. By shifting your perspective, you can use energy as a tool to unlock your potential.

Energy isn't simply about burning calories; it's about efficiently fueling your body. The way you manage energy balance—by aligning caloric intake with physical demands—can determine the speed and sustainability of your results. For instance, someone overeating while training for fat loss will struggle to see progress, while undereating during muscle-building phases can lead to fatigue and stalled growth. The source of your energy also matters. Foods rich in nutrients provide lasting energy, helping you push harder in workouts and recover faster. In contrast, empty calories from processed foods often leave you sluggish and unmotivated.

By understanding how energy impacts your body, you gain the ability to adjust your habits to match your goals. Whether through fine-tuning portion sizes or choosing whole, nutrient-dense foods, your choices shape how your body utilizes energy. This isn't just about achieving a specific aesthetic but also about feeling strong, energized, and capable every day. Recognizing the importance of energy shifts the focus from short-term fixes to a sustainable lifestyle that delivers long-term results.

Harnessing the power of energy balance transforms your fitness journey from a guessing game into a calculated, rewarding endeavor.

# The Quality of Calories

## 2.1 Nutrient-Dense Foods vs. Empty Calories: Highlight the Importance of Food Quality

Calories may measure energy, but not all calories are created equal. The quality of your food choices matters just as much as the quantity. Nutrient-dense foods, packed with vitamins, minerals, and essential nutrients, fuel your body for optimal performance. Empty calories, on the other hand, provide energy but little else, leaving your body undernourished and craving more.

Imagine two meals: one consists of grilled salmon, roasted vegetables, and quinoa, while the other is a slice of pizza and a soda. Both meals could have the same calorie count, but their effects on your body are worlds apart. The nutrient-dense meal provides protein for muscle repair, complex carbohydrates for sustained energy, and healthy fats for hormone support. Meanwhile, the pizza and soda deliver mostly refined carbs and unhealthy fats, causing energy crashes and providing minimal nourishment. Over time, relying on empty calories can lead to fatigue, weight gain, and deficiencies, while nutrient-dense foods promote vitality and long-term health.

The importance of food quality goes beyond physical benefits; it also impacts mental clarity, mood, and motivation. When you fuel your body with high-quality foods, you experience fewer energy slumps and greater focus, allowing you to stay consistent with your fitness goals. Conversely, empty calories often leave you feeling sluggish and unsatisfied, perpetuating unhealthy eating habits.

The path to better health begins with prioritizing whole, nutrient-dense foods. Think lean proteins like chicken, fish, and tofu; vibrant vegetables; whole grains like brown rice and oats; and healthy fats from avocados and nuts. By making these foods the foundation of your diet, you're not just counting calories—you're making every calorie count.

## 2.2 How Macro Distribution Impacts Energy: Connect Macros to Energy Levels

Understanding how macronutrients—protein, carbohydrates, and fats—affect energy can transform your approach to food. These three macros aren't just building blocks of nutrition; they're dynamic contributors to how your body feels and performs throughout the day.

Carbohydrates are your body's primary energy source, acting like high-octane fuel for workouts and daily activities. They're quickly converted to glucose, providing immediate energy. Without enough carbs, you may feel drained, struggle to complete workouts, and even compromise recovery. Protein, while often celebrated for muscle repair, also plays a role in energy stabilization. By slowing digestion, protein helps maintain steady energy levels and reduces mid-day crashes. Fats, often misunderstood, are crucial for long-lasting energy and are especially important for endurance activities. They also support brain health, keeping you mentally sharp.

The way you balance these macros determines your energy levels. For example, a breakfast rich in protein and healthy fats, like eggs and avocado, provides sustained energy and focus, perfect for a productive morning. A pre-workout meal with carbs, like oatmeal topped with fruit, ensures your body has the quick energy it needs to perform at its best. However, neglecting any macro or consuming them in unbalanced proportions can leave you feeling tired or bloated, hampering your goals.

The key lies in understanding your body's needs. Someone focused on fat loss may reduce carbs but still include enough to support workouts, while someone building muscle may increase protein and carbs. Experimenting with macro ratios and observing how your body responds allows you to optimize energy levels for both physical and mental performance.

## 2.3 Practical Meal Examples: Provide Real-Life Examples of Quality Meals

Knowing the theory of nutrition is one thing, but applying it to real life is what creates results. Crafting meals that balance quality calories and macronutrients can feel daunting, but with a little planning, it becomes second nature.

Start your day with a nutrient-dense breakfast to fuel your morning. A perfect example is a bowl of oatmeal topped with almond butter, chia seeds, and mixed berries. This meal combines complex carbs for sustained energy, healthy fats for satiety, and a hint of protein to keep hunger at bay. For lunch, consider a grilled chicken salad with mixed greens, quinoa, and a drizzle of olive oil. This dish delivers a well-rounded profile of lean protein, healthy fats, and fiber-packed carbs to keep you energized.

For a post-workout meal, think about a grilled salmon fillet paired with sweet potatoes and steamed broccoli. The salmon provides protein and omega-3 fats, while the sweet potatoes replenish glycogen stores, and broccoli offers a nutrient boost. Even snacks can contribute to your goals—Greek yogurt with a handful of nuts is an excellent mid-day option that balances protein and fats.

Dinner might include a turkey and vegetable stir-fry over brown rice. The turkey supplies lean protein, while the rice and vegetables offer a combination of energy and fiber. These meals not only nourish your body but also demonstrate how nutrient-dense foods can be delicious and satisfying.

Preparing meals in advance and keeping your pantry stocked with healthy staples ensures you're ready to make smart choices. By focusing on whole, nutrient-rich ingredients, you build meals that satisfy your hunger, energize your day, and support your goals, proving that quality calories are the foundation of a thriving, fit lifestyle.

# Applying the Science

## 3.1 Tracking Your Intake: Teach Effective Calorie and Macro Logging

The difference between guessing and knowing can make or break your fitness goals. Tracking your calorie and macro intake bridges that gap, giving you the clarity needed to achieve consistent results. While it might seem tedious at first, this habit transforms your relationship with food and puts you in control of your progress.

Tracking begins with understanding your personal caloric and macro needs, which depend on factors like age, weight, activity level, and fitness goals. Using tools like calorie calculators or apps such as MyFitnessPal can simplify the process. Once you've determined your target calories and macro ratios, you can begin logging everything you eat and drink throughout the day.

To track effectively, precision matters. Use a kitchen scale to measure portions, ensuring accuracy instead of relying on rough estimates. Reading food labels is essential, as it helps you break down calories and macros into usable data. For foods without labels, like fruits or cooked dishes, online databases provide reliable information. Consistency is key; logging even small bites or sips can reveal hidden calories that impact your progress.

Beyond just numbers, tracking also helps you identify patterns. Are you overeating carbs and under-consuming protein? Are your meals balanced or skewed toward processed options? These insights guide your adjustments, making tracking not just a tool but a roadmap to success. Over time, as you familiarize yourself with portion sizes and macro distribution, logging becomes second nature, empowering you to make informed choices even without an app in hand.

## 3.2 Avoiding Common Calorie Tracking Errors: Highlight Common Pitfalls

Tracking your intake is only effective if done correctly. Many fall into common traps that lead to frustration and stagnation. By identifying and avoiding these errors, you can ensure your efforts yield the desired results.

One of the most frequent mistakes is underestimating portion sizes. Without measuring, it's easy to assume a serving of rice or peanut butter is smaller than it is, resulting in untracked calories that add up over time. Another issue is neglecting to log "hidden calories" from cooking oils, condiments, and beverages. A splash of cream in your coffee or a drizzle of salad dressing may seem insignificant but can significantly impact your overall intake.

Relying solely on packaged food labels or restaurant estimates can also lead to inaccuracies. Labels allow for a margin of error, and restaurant dishes often contain more calories than advertised. When dining out, it's safer to overestimate portions rather than trust listed values. Emotional eating or binge episodes are another pitfall. Failing to log these instances not only skews your data but also disconnects you from the habit of accountability.

Finally, the all-or-nothing mindset can derail progress. Missing a day of tracking or slipping up on a meal doesn't mean your efforts are wasted. Instead of abandoning the practice, view setbacks as opportunities to learn. The goal is consistency, not perfection. By staying mindful and making small adjustments, you can avoid these pitfalls and maintain accurate, effective tracking.

## 3.3 Turning Theory into Practice: Share Practical Meal-Planning Steps

Understanding calories and macros is half the battle; the real challenge lies in implementing that knowledge into daily life. Practical meal planning bridges the gap between theory and action, simplifying your journey toward a healthier, more balanced diet.

Start by defining your goals and calorie requirements. Once you know how many calories and macros you need, divide them across your meals. For example, if you aim for 2,000 calories with a 40/30/30 macro split, you might allocate 800 calories for breakfast, 600 for lunch, 400 for dinner, and 200 for snacks. Breaking it down makes the process manageable and ensures you're nourishing your body consistently throughout the day.

When planning meals, prioritize whole, nutrient-dense foods. Build each plate around a lean protein source, such as chicken breast, tofu, or eggs, paired with a complex carbohydrate like quinoa or sweet potatoes, and add healthy fats from avocado or olive oil. Include colorful vegetables to boost fiber and micronutrient intake. The key is balance: every meal should provide fuel, repair, and satisfaction.

Batch cooking can save time and eliminate decision fatigue. Dedicate a few hours each week to preparing staples like grilled chicken, roasted veggies, and pre-measured snacks. Store them in portioned containers for easy access. This strategy not only keeps you on track but also minimizes the temptation of grabbing unhealthy options.

Flexibility is also essential. Life doesn't always adhere to plans, so learning to make smart choices on the go is invaluable. At restaurants, opt for grilled or baked dishes and ask for dressings and sauces on the side. If you indulge occasionally, balance it out by adjusting your next meal. Remember, consistency over time matters more than occasional deviations.

By incorporating these steps into your routine, you turn the science of calories and macros into actionable habits. Meal planning transforms from a chore into a strategy, empowering you to achieve your fitness goals while enjoying a sustainable, balanced lifestyle.

# Protein Power

## The Role of Protein

### 1.1 Why Protein is Key to Fitness Goals: Its Muscle-Building Role

Imagine sculpting your body into a masterpiece, each muscle defined and strong. The secret behind this transformation lies in a single nutrient: protein. Often hailed as the building block of life, protein plays a pivotal role in muscle development and overall fitness.

When you engage in resistance training or any strenuous activity, your muscle fibers experience microscopic tears. This might sound detrimental, but it's a natural and essential part of muscle growth. Protein comes into play by repairing these tiny tears, leading to increased muscle mass and strength. The amino acids derived from dietary protein are the fundamental components your body utilizes in this repair process. Without adequate protein intake, your muscles would struggle to recover, hindering progress toward your fitness goals.

Scientific research underscores the importance of protein in muscle synthesis. Studies indicate that individuals aiming to build muscle should consume more than the standard recommended dietary allowance. Specifically, an intake of 1.2 to 1.7 grams of protein per kilogram of body weight daily is beneficial for muscle growth. For athletes or those with highly active lifestyles, this requirement might be even higher, potentially up to 2.0 grams per kilogram.

However, it's not just about the quantity of protein but also the quality and timing. Incorporating high-quality protein sources such as lean meats, dairy, eggs, or plant-based options like legumes and tofu can provide the essential amino acids necessary for muscle repair. Additionally, distributing protein intake evenly throughout the day and consuming protein-rich meals or snacks post-workout can enhance muscle protein synthesis, optimizing recovery and growth.

In essence, protein is indispensable for anyone striving to achieve fitness milestones. It not only facilitates muscle repair and growth but also supports overall bodily functions, ensuring you have the strength and vitality to pursue your fitness journey. By prioritizing adequate and high-quality protein intake, you're laying a solid foundation for success in your health and fitness endeavors.

## 1.2 How Protein Affects Satiety: Managing Hunger with Protein

Consider the challenge of adhering to a diet while constantly battling hunger pangs. What if there was a way to feel fuller for longer, making it easier to manage your appetite and achieve your weight management goals? Enter protein—a nutrient renowned not only for its muscle-building properties but also for its remarkable ability to enhance satiety.

Satiety refers to the feeling of fullness and the suppression of hunger after eating. Among the three macronutrients—carbohydrates, fats, and proteins—protein has been found to be the most satiating. This means that meals rich in protein can lead to a greater sense of fullness, reducing overall calorie intake and aiding in weight management.

The mechanisms behind protein's satiating effects are multifaceted. Firstly, protein influences the release of appetite-regulating hormones. It stimulates the secretion of hormones such as peptide YY and GLP-1, both of which promote feelings of fullness. Simultaneously, protein intake can reduce levels of ghrelin, the hormone responsible for stimulating hunger.

Moreover, protein has a higher thermic effect compared to fats and carbohydrates. This means that the body expends more energy to digest, absorb, and metabolize protein, which can contribute to increased satiety and a reduction in subsequent calorie intake.

In practical terms, incorporating protein-rich foods into your diet can be a strategic approach to control hunger. Foods such as Greek yogurt, lean meats, legumes, and eggs are excellent choices. For instance, studies have shown that consuming yogurt as a high-protein snack can improve appetite control and reduce subsequent food intake in healthy women.

It's also worth noting that the timing of protein intake can influence satiety. Starting your day with a protein-rich breakfast can lead to reduced hunger throughout the day, potentially decreasing the likelihood of overeating during later meals.

Protein plays a crucial role in hunger management. By enhancing feelings of fullness through hormonal regulation and increased energy expenditure during digestion, protein can be a valuable ally in controlling appetite and supporting weight management efforts. Incorporating adequate amounts of high-quality protein into your daily diet can make the journey toward your health and fitness goals more attainable and sustainable.

## Setting Your Protein Intake

## 2.1 Daily Protein Requirements by Goal: Defining Your Protein Needs

Understanding how much protein you need daily is fundamental to achieving your health and fitness goals. Your protein requirements largely depend on whether you're aiming to build muscle, lose weight, or maintain your current physique. Each of these goals calls for a specific approach to protein intake.

For those pursuing muscle gain, consuming adequate protein is critical to repairing and building muscle tissue. When engaging in resistance training, your body requires more protein to support recovery and growth. Research highlights that individuals seeking muscle growth should aim for 1.2 to 2.0 grams of protein per kilogram of body weight daily. For instance, a 75-kilogram individual needs approximately 90 to 150 grams of protein per day to optimize muscle synthesis.

If weight loss is your goal, protein serves a dual purpose. It not only helps preserve lean muscle mass while shedding fat but also plays a significant role in controlling hunger. A diet higher in protein can make calorie restriction more manageable, as protein enhances satiety. For effective weight loss, experts recommend consuming around 1.2 to 1.5 grams of protein per kilogram of body weight daily. A person weighing 70 kilograms, for example, would need 84 to 105 grams of protein.

For those focused on maintaining their current body weight and overall health, the general guideline is an intake of 0.8 grams of protein per kilogram of body weight. However, for active individuals or those with higher energy demands, slightly increasing this to 1.0 gram per kilogram can support muscle repair and daily activity. A 65-kilogram person aiming for maintenance would therefore require 52 to 65 grams of protein daily.

These recommendations provide a starting point, but individual factors such as age, gender, and activity level can influence your protein needs. Consulting with a healthcare professional can help you determine the ideal amount for your specific lifestyle and objectives. The key to success lies in aligning your protein intake with your goals, ensuring your body has the nutrients it needs to thrive.

## 2.2 Finding Protein in Everyday Foods: Common Protein Sources

Incorporating adequate protein into your diet doesn't have to be complicated or expensive. Everyday foods offer a variety of rich and accessible protein sources that can seamlessly fit into your routine, whether you prefer animal-based or plant-based options.

Animal-based proteins are among the most complete sources, providing all the essential amino acids your body needs. Lean meats like chicken, turkey, and beef are excellent options for boosting your intake. For instance, a single serving of cooked chicken breast offers about 31 grams of protein, making it a staple for those aiming to meet higher daily requirements. Similarly, seafood such as salmon and shrimp provides not only protein but also heart-healthy omega-3 fatty acids. Dairy products like milk, yogurt, and cheese contribute significantly to daily protein intake while also offering the added benefit of calcium.

For individuals seeking plant-based alternatives, protein-rich foods like beans, lentils, and chickpeas are excellent choices. A cup of cooked lentils, for example, contains about 18 grams of protein and is versatile enough to be included in soups, salads, or side dishes. Soy products such as tofu and tempeh are also highly adaptable and packed with protein. Meanwhile, whole grains like quinoa provide both protein and essential nutrients like fiber, making them a valuable addition to meals.

The beauty of these options lies in their accessibility and adaptability. From grilled chicken to a quinoa salad with roasted vegetables, these protein-rich foods can be incorporated into meals that suit your lifestyle, dietary preferences, and fitness goals.

## 2.3 Balancing Protein Across Meals: Tips for Even Distribution

While meeting your total daily protein goal is crucial, how you distribute protein across your meals can significantly impact your results. Research shows that evenly spreading protein intake throughout the day can enhance muscle protein synthesis and help manage hunger effectively.

Starting your day with a protein-rich breakfast sets the tone for balanced eating. A meal that includes eggs, Greek yogurt, or a protein smoothie not only provides a strong nutritional foundation but also helps curb mid-morning hunger. Consistently including protein at lunch and dinner can further stabilize energy levels and support muscle repair. For example, a balanced lunch featuring a serving of chicken or tofu paired with vegetables and whole grains ensures you're meeting your nutritional needs.

Even snacks can be an opportunity to boost your protein intake. Options like a handful of nuts, a slice of cheese, or a serving of hummus with vegetables offer a quick and satisfying way to bridge the gap between meals. By incorporating these snacks strategically, you can maintain steady energy and stave off cravings.

Finally, meal planning plays a vital role in achieving an even distribution of protein. Preparing meals in advance allows you to ensure that every plate contains a balanced portion of protein, carbohydrates, and healthy fats. By prioritizing protein at every meal and snack, you'll maximize its benefits, ensuring your body has the consistent fuel it needs to build muscle, regulate appetite, and achieve your health goals.

# Protein Hacks for Busy Men

## 3.1 Quick and Easy Protein Sources: Convenient Options for Busy Lives

In the fast-paced world we live in, finding time to prepare protein-rich meals can be challenging. However, there are plenty of quick and easy protein sources that ensure you stay on track with your nutrition goals without sacrificing time or convenience.

One of the simplest and quickest protein options is Greek yogurt. A single serving can contain up to 20 grams of protein, and it's ready to eat right out of the container. For a filling snack or breakfast, you can pair it with some nuts, seeds, or fruit for a balanced meal. Similarly, eggs are a versatile and fast protein source. Whether you scramble them, make an omelet, or even boil them in advance, eggs provide high-quality protein and essential nutrients. One large egg contains around 6 grams of protein and can be eaten on its own or added to other meals.

For even quicker solutions, protein bars or shakes can come to the rescue. Many protein bars offer a convenient and portable option that provides anywhere from 15 to 30 grams of protein, depending on the brand. The same goes for protein shakes, which can be mixed in seconds and consumed on the go. For those who prefer to avoid processed products, canned tuna or salmon is another quick protein-packed food. A single can often contains 25 grams or more of protein and can be added to a salad, sandwich, or eaten straight from the can.

Frozen protein-rich meals or ingredients can also be a lifesaver. Items like frozen chicken breasts, pre-cooked shrimp, or frozen edamame can be heated quickly and incorporated into a variety of meals. These options save time without compromising the quality of your protein intake.

# 3.2 Affordable Protein Options: Budget-Friendly Sources

Eating enough protein doesn't have to break the bank. There are plenty of affordable protein sources that provide excellent nutritional value while keeping your grocery bill low.

One of the most budget-friendly protein options is beans and lentils. These plant-based proteins are not only inexpensive but also rich in fiber, making them an excellent choice for both protein and overall health. A bag of dried lentils or beans costs very little, and you can prepare large batches that last for several meals. A cup of cooked lentils can offer up to 18 grams of protein, providing a filling and cost-effective solution.

Canned tuna and other canned fish options are also incredibly affordable and protein-dense. A can of tuna typically provides around 25 grams of protein for just a few dollars. This makes it an excellent choice for those on a tight budget who still want to meet their protein needs.

Chicken is another versatile and affordable protein source. While premium cuts can be expensive, bone-in, skinless chicken thighs or chicken legs are typically more budget-friendly and still provide ample protein. Ground turkey is another option that offers great value, often priced lower than beef, and can be used in a wide range of meals, from chili to stir-fries.

For a plant-based approach, tofu and tempeh offer affordable protein options as well. Both are made from soybeans and provide a good amount of protein for their price. A block of tofu typically contains around 10 to 15 grams of protein per serving and can be used in countless recipes.

Incorporating a combination of these budget-friendly sources into your meals can help you meet your daily protein requirements without stretching your budget too thin.

# 3.3 Meal Prep for Protein Success: Simplifying Protein Prep for Busy Schedules

When time is limited, meal prep becomes a game-changer, especially for ensuring you hit your protein targets throughout the week. By dedicating a small amount of time once or twice a week to meal prepping, you can have protein-rich meals ready to go, reducing the temptation to skip meals or resort to unhealthy snacks.

Start by selecting protein-rich foods that can be cooked in bulk and stored for later use. Cooking a large batch of chicken breasts, ground turkey, or lean beef can provide you with the base for several meals. Once cooked, these proteins can be portioned out into individual servings, making it easy to grab and go throughout the week. Similarly, cooking a large pot of beans or lentils can ensure you always have a plant-based protein source on hand.

When preparing your protein, consider also incorporating a variety of vegetables and whole grains to create well-rounded meals. For example, you can prepare quinoa or rice in bulk, and pair it with grilled chicken and roasted vegetables. Store these meals in individual containers for easy access. Another great option for meal prep is batch-making protein-packed salads with grilled chicken, beans, and seeds. These salads can last for several days in the fridge and can be paired with a variety of dressings for different flavors.

For even more convenience, consider using a slow cooker or Instant Pot to prepare large quantities of protein-rich meals with minimal effort. These appliances allow you to throw ingredients in, set them, and let them cook while you focus on other tasks. For instance, you can slow-cook a beef stew or chicken chili packed with protein, and portion it out for several days.

Incorporating protein into meal prep ensures that you always have nutritious, protein-rich meals ready, regardless of how busy your schedule is. Whether it's pre-cooked chicken, homemade protein bars, or bulk-cooked beans, meal prepping saves you time and helps you stick to your goals.

44

# Carbs: Friend or Foe

## Understanding Carbohydrates

### 1.1 Carbs as the Body's Energy Source

Imagine a car without fuel—it may have a powerful engine and sleek design, but it's going nowhere. That's how your body operates without carbohydrates. These macronutrients are your body's primary energy source, fueling everything from your heartbeat to your most intense workouts. Every movement you make, every thought you think, requires energy. Carbs provide that energy in the form of glucose, which your body either uses immediately or stores for later in the form of glycogen.

When you consume carbs, enzymes in your digestive system break them down into glucose molecules. This glucose enters your bloodstream and powers your cells. During high-intensity activities—like running or weightlifting—your body relies heavily on these glycogen stores. Unlike fats or proteins, which take longer to convert to energy, carbs are a fast and efficient source of fuel.

But what happens when you skip carbs? Your body shifts to burning fat and even protein for energy, a process called ketosis. While this can be beneficial for specific goals like weight loss, it may not support peak performance in physical activities. Carbs are essential for optimal brain function, muscle recovery, and even hormone regulation. It's not about labeling them as "good" or "bad" but understanding how they support your body's complex systems.

Neglecting carbs can lead to fatigue, poor mental clarity, and decreased physical endurance. On the flip side, overindulging, especially in processed carbs, can result in weight gain and insulin resistance. The key lies in balance. As the body's energy currency, carbohydrates are indispensable—but using them wisely is your blueprint for building a better body.

## 1.2 Types of Carbs: Simple vs. Complex

Not all carbs are created equal, and understanding the difference between simple and complex carbohydrates is pivotal. Simple carbs, like those found in candy, soda, and pastries, are quickly digested and cause a rapid spike in blood sugar. These "sugar rushes" are fleeting and often leave you feeling drained.

In contrast, complex carbs are like slow-burning logs on a fire. Found in whole grains, vegetables, and legumes, these carbs provide a steady, prolonged release of energy. Their molecular structure—made of longer chains of sugar molecules—takes your body longer to break down. This results in stabilized blood sugar levels and sustained energy.

Fiber, a key component of many complex carbs, plays an additional role. It slows digestion, promotes gut health, and helps you feel full longer. Foods rich in fiber, like oats and brown rice, deliver both energy and essential nutrients, such as vitamins and minerals.

The real challenge comes with navigating the modern diet. Processed foods often blur the line between simple and complex carbs, sneaking in added sugars while stripping away fiber. The glycemic index—a measure of how quickly a food spikes your blood sugar—is a helpful tool for making informed choices. For example, a piece of white bread has a high glycemic index, while whole grain bread has a much lower one, offering more stable energy.

By focusing on complex carbs and minimizing processed sugars, you can transform your diet into a steady energy source. It's not about demonizing sugar or glorifying grains but recognizing the different ways they impact your body. Complex carbs are the cornerstone of a sustainable and healthy lifestyle, equipping you with the energy and nutrients to thrive.

## 1.3 How Carbs Impact Performance

Carbs are not just about energy—they are the secret weapon for maximizing athletic performance. When you engage in intense physical activity, your muscles rely on glycogen, the stored form of glucose, for quick bursts of power. Without enough carbs, those glycogen stores deplete rapidly, leaving you fatigued and unable to perform at your best.

Pre-workout meals rich in carbs act like a top-off for your glycogen reserves. Whether it's a bowl of oatmeal or a banana, these foods prepare your body for endurance and strength. During the activity itself, especially if it's long or grueling, consuming carbs can prevent the dreaded energy crash.

Post-workout, the role of carbs shifts from fuel to recovery. They help replenish glycogen stores and facilitate muscle repair, especially when paired with protein. A smoothie with a mix of fruits and protein powder can be an excellent recovery option.

On the flip side, insufficient carb intake can hinder progress. Athletes on low-carb diets often report reduced stamina and slower recovery times. This doesn't mean everyone needs the same amount of carbs; your intake should match your activity level and goals. A marathon runner will require more carbs than someone focusing on light yoga.

Scientific studies underline carbs' pivotal role in physical performance. They highlight how high-carb diets improve endurance athletes' performance while balanced carb consumption supports strength training and muscle gains. To achieve peak performance, you need to think of carbs not as optional but as essential tools in your fitness arsenal.

By aligning your carbohydrate intake with your energy demands, you unlock your body's full potential. It's about fueling with intention, understanding that the right carbs at the right time can elevate your workouts and expedite recovery. In the pursuit of your best body, carbs are not just a friend—they're an indispensable ally.

# Customizing Carb Intake

## 2.1 Carb Needs by Activity Level

Carbohydrate intake isn't a one-size-fits-all equation; it varies greatly depending on your activity level. The more energy you expend, the more carbs your body requires to sustain performance and recovery. Think of carbs as your body's fuel tank—low activity levels demand smaller tanks, while high-intensity workouts require a full reservoir.

For sedentary individuals or those with light activity levels, such as walking or yoga, the body requires fewer carbohydrates. In this case, focusing on nutrient-dense, low-glycemic carbs like vegetables and whole grains ensures sustained energy without unnecessary calorie surplus. On the other hand, moderate activity levels, like regular gym sessions or recreational sports, call for a moderate intake. Here, including starchy carbs like sweet potatoes or quinoa provides the balance of fuel and nutrients your body needs.

When it comes to athletes or individuals engaging in intense physical activity, the demand skyrockets. High-intensity training depletes glycogen stores rapidly, making adequate carb intake essential. In these cases, consuming fast-digesting carbs, such as fruits or even sports drinks during workouts, ensures energy levels remain high.

The science behind this is straightforward: carbohydrates are the body's most efficient energy source, and failing to match intake to activity can result in fatigue, poor performance, and even muscle breakdown. However, overloading on carbs when your activity levels are low can lead to weight gain and insulin resistance.

By aligning your carb intake with your activity level, you give your body exactly what it needs—nothing more, nothing less. Understanding this balance is key to optimizing your energy, enhancing recovery, and avoiding the pitfalls of under- or over-fueling.

## 2.2 Timing Your Carb Consumption

When it comes to carbohydrates, timing can be as crucial as quantity. Consuming carbs at the right times can maximize their benefits and align them with your fitness goals, whether it's enhancing performance, boosting recovery, or improving body composition.

Pre-workout carbs play an essential role in fueling your training sessions. Eating a meal rich in complex carbohydrates, such as oatmeal or whole-grain toast, about 1–3 hours before exercise provides a steady release of energy. If you're short on time, a quick-digesting option like a banana or a small smoothie 30 minutes before a workout can be equally effective.

Intra-workout carbs, often in the form of easily digestible sugars, become critical during prolonged or high-intensity sessions. They help sustain energy levels, delay fatigue, and improve performance. For endurance athletes, sipping on a carbohydrate-based drink can be a game-changer.

Post-workout, the focus shifts to recovery. Consuming carbs within 30 minutes of finishing exercise helps replenish glycogen stores and jumpstarts the muscle repair process. Pairing carbs with protein, such as a recovery shake or a turkey sandwich, optimizes these benefits.

For general energy management, spreading carb intake throughout the day is vital. Starting your day with a balanced breakfast that includes complex carbs sets the tone, while mid-day meals ensure consistent energy levels. Evening carb consumption, often debated, can be beneficial for recovery and sleep, especially after evening workouts.

Timing carbs strategically allows you to harness their full potential, making them work with your goals rather than against them. Whether it's fueling performance or speeding up recovery, knowing when to consume carbs can make all the difference.

## 2.3 Adjusting Carbs for Fat Loss or Muscle Gain

Carbohydrates play a pivotal role in both fat loss and muscle gain, but how you consume them depends entirely on your specific goals. Adjusting your carb intake strategically can help you tilt the scales in your favor, whether you're aiming to shed body fat or pack on lean muscle.

For fat loss, the key lies in creating a calorie deficit while maintaining enough carbs to fuel your workouts and daily activities. Reducing carb intake slightly—particularly from refined sugars and processed foods—can lower overall calorie consumption while stabilizing blood sugar levels. This doesn't mean cutting carbs entirely; doing so can lead to energy crashes and muscle loss. Instead, prioritize complex carbs, such as vegetables, legumes, and whole grains, which provide lasting energy and keep hunger at bay.

In contrast, muscle gain requires a calorie surplus, and carbohydrates are a crucial component. High-quality carbs provide the energy needed for intense workouts and create the anabolic environment necessary for muscle growth. Incorporating carb sources like rice, potatoes, and fruits around your workouts maximizes glycogen replenishment and supports muscle recovery.

Cycling carbs—alternating high and low intake days—can be an effective strategy for both goals. High-carb days fuel intense training and recovery, while low-carb days encourage fat burning. This approach keeps your metabolism flexible and responsive.

Ultimately, the success of either goal depends on balance and consistency. Extreme carb restrictions or overindulgence can backfire, leading to stagnation or unwanted weight changes. By customizing your carb intake to match your objectives, you can create a tailored nutrition plan that supports sustainable progress. Whether it's fat loss or muscle gain, the right carb strategy is the cornerstone of achieving your best body.

# Smart Carb Choices

## 3.1 Best Carb Sources for Performance

When it comes to carbs, quality matters just as much as quantity. Choosing the right sources can enhance your physical performance, boost recovery, and sustain energy levels throughout the day. High-quality carbohydrates are nutrient-dense, providing not only energy but also essential vitamins, minerals, and fiber.

For athletes or anyone leading an active lifestyle, whole grains are a top choice. Brown rice, quinoa, oats, and whole-grain bread are complex carbs that release energy slowly, keeping you fueled for longer periods. They also contain B vitamins, which are vital for energy metabolism. Sweet potatoes and other starchy vegetables, such as butternut squash and beets, offer a combination of carbohydrates and antioxidants, making them excellent pre- or post-workout options.

Fruits, another high-quality source, are nature's convenient energy snack. Bananas, for example, are packed with easily digestible carbs and potassium, perfect for pre-workout fueling. Apples, oranges, and berries provide fiber along with natural sugars, delivering a sustained energy boost without causing blood sugar spikes.

Legumes, like lentils, chickpeas, and black beans, deserve a spot on your plate. They are not only rich in complex carbs but also packed with protein and fiber, making them ideal for both performance and satiety. Additionally, they have a low glycemic index, meaning they won't cause sharp blood sugar fluctuations.

For those needing rapid energy replenishment during or after workouts, low-fiber carbs like white rice or ripe bananas can be beneficial. These options are quickly absorbed and can kickstart glycogen restoration when timing is critical.

Ultimately, the best carb sources are minimally processed and nutrient-rich, supporting both energy and recovery. By incorporating a variety of these foods into your diet, you can maximize performance while keeping your body nourished.

## 3.2 Avoiding Processed Carbs

Processed carbs are everywhere—from the breakfast cereals lining grocery store shelves to the pastries tempting you at coffee shops. While they might taste good and offer quick energy, their long-term effects on your health and performance can be detrimental. Understanding why and how to avoid processed carbs is a key step toward smarter carb choices.

Processed carbs are typically stripped of their natural fiber, vitamins, and minerals during manufacturing. Foods like white bread, sugary snacks, and packaged desserts fall into this category. When consumed, these products lead to rapid blood sugar spikes followed by crashes, leaving you feeling sluggish and hungry again soon after. Over time, a diet high in processed carbs can contribute to weight gain, insulin resistance, and chronic health conditions like type 2 diabetes.

Healthier alternatives are abundant and far more satisfying. Instead of white bread, choose whole-grain or sprouted bread, which retains its fiber and nutrients. Swap sugary cereals for oatmeal topped with fresh fruits and nuts. Craving a snack? Replace chips with air-popped popcorn or homemade sweet potato wedges. These swaps retain the flavor and convenience while supporting your body's energy needs.

Reading food labels is another effective strategy. Look out for hidden sugars and refined grains listed as ingredients. Opt for foods with whole, recognizable ingredients and minimal additives. The closer a food is to its natural state, the better it is for you.

Avoiding processed carbs doesn't mean you have to eliminate all indulgences. It's about making intentional choices that align with your goals. By prioritizing whole, unprocessed carbs, you'll find yourself with more energy, fewer cravings, and better performance overall.

## 3.3 Building a Carb-Friendly Meal

Crafting a balanced, carb-friendly meal is easier than it might seem. The key is combining high-quality carbs with protein, healthy fats, and plenty of vegetables to create a plate that satisfies your taste buds and fuels your body.

Start with a foundation of complex carbohydrates. For instance, choose a base of quinoa or brown rice. These grains provide sustained energy and pair well with a variety of flavors. For a lower-carb option, consider roasted sweet potatoes or a bed of leafy greens like spinach or kale.

Next, add a source of lean protein to balance the meal and support muscle repair. Grilled chicken, baked salmon, or plant-based options like tofu or lentils work perfectly. Protein helps slow the digestion of carbs, ensuring a steady release of energy throughout the day.

Healthy fats complete the meal and enhance nutrient absorption. Add a dollop of guacamole, a drizzle of olive oil, or a sprinkle of chopped nuts or seeds. These fats not only improve the meal's texture but also keep you feeling full and satisfied.

Finally, pile on non-starchy vegetables for added volume and nutrients. Roasted broccoli, sautéed bell peppers, or fresh cucumber slices add vibrant colors and crunch. These veggies are low in calories but high in fiber and antioxidants, making them the ideal complement to your carb-friendly meal.

For example, a balanced dinner could be grilled salmon served over quinoa, topped with a handful of arugula, and drizzled with lemon-tahini dressing. On the side, enjoy roasted sweet potato wedges and steamed asparagus.

Building meals like this ensures you're making the most of your carbohydrate intake while supporting your body's energy and recovery needs. A carb-friendly meal isn't just about carbs—it's about harmony among all nutrients to create a plate that's as nourishing as it is delicious.

# Fats That Fuel

## The Importance of Dietary Fats

### 1.1 How Fats Support Hormones and Brain Health

Imagine your body as a finely tuned orchestra, with each instrument playing a crucial role in creating harmonious health. Dietary fats are the masterful conductors, orchestrating vital functions that keep your body in perfect rhythm.

Fats are indispensable for hormone production. Hormones act as the body's chemical messengers, regulating processes from metabolism to mood. Without adequate fat intake, the synthesis of essential hormones like estrogen and testosterone can be compromised, leading to imbalances that affect everything from energy levels to reproductive health. In fact, certain fats are precursors to hormones, meaning they are the building blocks necessary for hormone creation. This underscores the importance of including healthy fats in your diet to maintain hormonal harmony.

Beyond hormonal health, fats are vital for brain function. The human brain is composed of nearly 60% fat, emphasizing the need for dietary fats to maintain its structure and function. Omega-3 fatty acids, a type of polyunsaturated fat, are particularly crucial. They contribute to the fluidity of cell membranes in the brain, facilitating efficient communication between neurons. This enhances cognitive functions such as memory, focus, and learning. Moreover, omega-3s have anti-inflammatory properties that protect the brain against neurodegenerative diseases like Alzheimer's. A diet rich in these fats can therefore support long-term brain health and cognitive vitality.

In addition to their roles in hormone production and brain health, dietary fats aid in the absorption of fat-soluble vitamins—A, D, E, and K. These vitamins are essential for processes like vision, bone health, and immune function. Without sufficient fat intake, your body may struggle to absorb these nutrients, potentially leading to deficiencies. Therefore, incorporating healthy fats into your meals not only supports hormonal and brain health but also ensures you receive the full spectrum of benefits from your diet.

Incorporating healthy fats into your diet is not just beneficial but essential. Foods rich in unsaturated fats, such as avocados, nuts, and olive oil, provide the necessary components for hormone production and brain function. Fatty fish like salmon and mackerel are excellent sources of omega-3 fatty acids, further supporting cognitive health. By making conscious choices to include these fats in your meals, you empower your body to perform at its best, maintaining hormonal balance and cognitive sharpness.

## 1.2 Types of Fats: Good vs. Bad

In the vast landscape of nutrition, not all fats are created equal. Understanding the distinction between healthy and unhealthy fats is pivotal for making informed dietary choices that promote overall well-being.

**Healthy Fats:**

*1. Monounsaturated Fats*: These fats are liquid at room temperature and are known to improve blood cholesterol levels, reducing the risk of heart disease.

They are predominantly found in plant-based oils such as olive oil, as well as in avocados, nuts, and seeds. Incorporating monounsaturated fats into your diet can aid in maintaining healthy cholesterol levels and provide essential nutrients.

**2. *Polyunsaturated Fats:*** This category includes omega-3 and omega-6 fatty acids, which are essential fats that the body cannot produce on its own. Omega-3s, found in fatty fish like salmon, flaxseeds, and walnuts, play a crucial role in brain function and have anti-inflammatory properties. Omega-6s, present in oils such as soybean and sunflower oil, are important for growth and development. However, it's essential to maintain a balanced intake of omega-6 and omega-3 fatty acids to support overall health.

**Unhealthy Fats:**

**1. *Saturated Fats*:** Typically solid at room temperature, saturated fats are found in animal products like red meat, butter, and full-fat dairy. High intake of saturated fats can raise LDL (bad) cholesterol levels, increasing the risk of heart disease and stroke. Health organizations recommend limiting saturated fat intake to less than 10% of total daily calories to maintain heart health.

**2. *Trans Fats*:** These are the most detrimental fats, often found in partially hydrogenated oils used in processed and fried foods. Trans fats not only raise LDL cholesterol but also lower HDL (good) cholesterol, significantly elevating the risk of cardiovascular diseases. Due to their adverse health effects, many regulatory agencies have implemented measures to reduce trans fat content in foods.

Making conscious choices to replace unhealthy fats with healthy ones can have profound health benefits. For instance, swapping butter (high in saturated fat) with olive oil (rich in monounsaturated fat) can improve cholesterol levels and reduce heart disease risk. Similarly, choosing fatty fish over red meat provides beneficial omega-3s while reducing saturated fat intake. By understanding the types of fats and their impacts on health, you can tailor your diet to support cardiovascular health, enhance brain function, and maintain overall wellness.

## 1.3 Common Misconceptions About Fats

In the quest for a healthier lifestyle, dietary fats have often been misunderstood and unfairly vilified. Dispelling these misconceptions is essential for embracing a balanced diet that truly supports your health goals.

### 1: All Fats Lead to Weight Gain

Many people believe that consuming fats directly contributes to weight gain. While it's true that fats are calorie-dense—providing 9 calories per gram compared to 4 calories per gram for proteins and carbohydrates—they are also highly satiating. Healthy fats, such as those found in avocados, nuts, and olive oil, promote fullness and can help regulate appetite. This satiating effect may actually reduce overall calorie consumption. Additionally, the body uses dietary fats for energy, hormone production, and cell repair, making them a crucial part of a well-rounded diet. Simply put, not all fats are created equal, and their role in weight management is more nuanced than popular myths suggest.

### 2: Low-Fat Diets Are the Healthiest

The rise of low-fat diets in the 1980s and 1990s has ingrained the idea that eating less fat automatically equals better health. However, this oversimplification has led many people to replace fats with highly processed carbohydrates and sugars, which can contribute to weight gain and metabolic disorders. Research now shows that diets emphasizing healthy fats—such as the Mediterranean diet—can reduce the risk of heart disease, improve brain function, and even aid in weight management. Instead of fearing fats, the focus should be on choosing the right kinds in the correct amounts.

## 3: Cholesterol from Fats Is Always Harmful

The belief that all dietary fats raise cholesterol levels and increase heart disease risk is another widespread myth. While trans fats and excessive saturated fats can negatively impact cholesterol, unsaturated fats have the opposite effect. For example, omega-3 fatty acids found in fatty fish and walnuts can reduce inflammation and improve heart health. Additionally, recent research has shifted the focus from total cholesterol levels to the balance between HDL (good cholesterol) and LDL (bad cholesterol). Healthy fats support this balance, contributing to overall cardiovascular health.

## 4: Fat Is Unnecessary if You're Active

Some fitness enthusiasts think they can skip fats because they rely on carbs and protein for energy and muscle building. However, fats are essential for endurance athletes and active individuals alike. They provide a concentrated energy source, particularly during prolonged activities when glycogen stores are depleted. Moreover, fats aid in recovery by reducing inflammation and supporting joint health.

Understanding the truth about dietary fats can transform the way you approach your nutrition. By debunking these common myths, you'll realize that fats are not the enemy. Instead, they are vital allies in achieving optimal health, supporting hormone production, brain function, and overall well-being. Replacing fear with knowledge empowers you to make informed choices, integrating healthy fats into your diet while avoiding the pitfalls of misinformation.

# Incorporating Fats

## 2.1 How Much Fat Do You Need?

Fats are a vital macronutrient that plays an essential role in overall health, but like all things, balance is key. The amount of fat you should consume depends on several factors, such as your age, activity level, and health goals. General dietary guidelines recommend that fats make up about 20-35% of your total daily calories. For someone consuming a 2,000-calorie diet, this would translate to approximately 44-78 grams of fat per day. However, these numbers are not one-size-fits-all, and individual needs may vary depending on specific goals like weight management or muscle building.

While fats provide a concentrated source of energy, they also play a critical role in supporting the body's cellular structure, hormone production, and nutrient absorption. The challenge lies in ensuring that the types of fats you consume are the right ones. Unsaturated fats, including monounsaturated and polyunsaturated fats, should make up the majority of your fat intake, while saturated fats should be limited to less than 10% of your daily caloric intake. Trans fats, found in processed and fried foods, should be completely avoided, as they contribute to heart disease and other health issues.

It's also important to note that fats are calorie-dense, which means portion control is essential. Even healthy fats like those found in nuts and oils can quickly add up if consumed in excess. Therefore, while it's important to include fats in your diet, paying attention to portion sizes ensures they support rather than hinder your overall health goals.

## 2.2 Healthy Fat Sources

Incorporating fats into your diet can be both easy and delicious when you choose the right sources. Healthy fats come from a variety of whole food options, offering not just flavor but also essential nutrients that the body needs for proper functioning. Plant-based fats, such as those found in avocados, nuts, seeds, and oils like olive oil, are excellent sources of monounsaturated fats, which support heart health and contribute to healthy cholesterol levels. Avocados, for instance, are packed with fiber, potassium, and healthy fats, making them a perfect addition to meals or snacks.

Fatty fish like salmon, mackerel, and sardines are another top source of healthy fats, particularly omega-3 fatty acids. Omega-3s are crucial for brain health, reducing inflammation, and supporting cardiovascular health. Including fatty fish in your diet just a couple of times a week can significantly boost your intake of these beneficial fats.

While plant-based fats are generally favored for their health benefits, certain animal-based fats can also provide nutritional value. For example, eggs, particularly from pasture-raised chickens, are a great source of omega-3 fatty acids and provide high-quality protein. Additionally, full-fat dairy products like Greek yogurt and cheese can be part of a balanced diet, offering a mix of fats, protein, and essential vitamins and minerals.

For those who struggle to include enough fats from whole foods, omega-3 supplements or fortified foods like enriched eggs can be helpful. However, relying on whole food sources should always be the priority to maximize nutrient absorption and overall health benefits.

## 2.3 Balancing Fats in Your Diet

Incorporating fats into your daily routine requires more than just adding a few extra ingredients to your meals—it's about achieving the right balance. The goal is to include a variety of fats while ensuring they fit proportionally within your overall nutrient intake. To do this, it's important to prioritize unsaturated fats, such as those from olive oil, nuts, and fatty fish, while minimizing the consumption of saturated fats, which are often found in fatty meats and processed foods.

One way to achieve balance is by making simple swaps in your cooking. For example, replacing butter or margarine with olive oil or avocado oil can reduce saturated fat intake while boosting the intake of healthy fats. Similarly, opting for leaner cuts of meat or plant-based protein sources can help keep your overall fat intake in check. When cooking, it's important to pay attention to the oils you use, as some, like flaxseed or walnut oil, are best reserved for cold dishes due to their low smoke points.

Avoiding trans fats is also a key component of a balanced fat intake. These fats, often found in processed and fast foods, should be eliminated from your diet altogether. Trans fats not only raise bad cholesterol (LDL) but also lower good cholesterol (HDL), increasing the risk of heart disease and other chronic health issues.

Finally, balancing fats with other macronutrients, such as carbohydrates and proteins, is essential for maintaining a well-rounded diet. Healthy fats should complement other nutrient-dense foods, ensuring you're getting a variety of vitamins, minerals, and antioxidants. This approach ensures that fats aren't overconsumed at the expense of other nutrients, and helps maintain a sustainable and balanced eating pattern that supports long-term health.

By focusing on the types of fats you consume and their proportion in your diet, you can maximize the health benefits of fats while avoiding excesses that may lead to unwanted weight gain or health risks. Ultimately, a balanced diet that includes healthy fats in moderation, alongside carbohydrates and proteins, will support optimal energy levels, brain function, and overall well-being.

# Practical Fat Tips

## 3.1 Cooking with Fats

Cooking with fats doesn't have to be complicated, and when done right, it can significantly enhance the flavor and nutritional value of your meals. Healthy fats, in particular, provide essential fatty acids and help the body absorb fat-soluble vitamins like A, D, E, and K. The key is to choose the right fats for different cooking methods and make the most of their benefits.

When preparing meals, start by choosing fats that are stable at higher temperatures. For high-heat cooking like frying or sautéing, opt for oils with a high smoke point, such as avocado oil or grapeseed oil. These oils maintain their integrity and don't break down into harmful compounds at high temperatures. On the other hand, delicate oils like flaxseed, walnut, or hemp oil are best reserved for cold dishes, such as salad dressings or drizzling over roasted vegetables.

Olive oil is a versatile option that works well for medium-heat cooking and is perfect for dressings or as a drizzle on cooked dishes. Extra virgin olive oil, in particular, contains beneficial antioxidants and polyphenols, which support heart health. When sautéing vegetables or stir-frying, use a moderate amount of olive oil to bring out the natural flavors of your ingredients while enhancing their nutrient absorption.

For baking, you can use coconut oil, which offers a subtle flavor and a good balance of healthy saturated fats. When using oils for baking, however, be mindful of the quantities, as fats are calorie-dense. Incorporating healthy fats into cooking helps you maintain a balanced intake while enhancing the taste and nutrition of your meals.

Remember, the goal isn't to overdo fats, but to use them strategically to complement the overall nutrient profile of your dishes. Healthy fats can transform an ordinary meal into a flavorful, nourishing experience while supporting your body's nutritional needs.

## 3.2 Snacking on Healthy Fats

Snacking can be a great opportunity to add healthy fats into your diet, especially when you're on the go or need an energy boost between meals. However, it's essential to choose snacks that not only provide a satisfying taste but also contribute to your health goals without derailing your progress.

Nuts and seeds are some of the easiest and most portable sources of healthy fats. Almonds, walnuts, cashews, chia seeds, and flaxseeds are packed with monounsaturated and polyunsaturated fats, along with fiber and protein. A handful of mixed nuts can help curb hunger and provide lasting energy, keeping you satisfied until your next meal. Just be cautious with portion sizes, as nuts are calorie-dense. Pre-portioning snacks into small servings helps prevent overconsumption.

Another great option for a healthy fat snack is avocados. Their creamy texture and high content of monounsaturated fats make them perfect for spreading on whole-grain toast or for adding to salads. If you're looking for a quick snack, simply slice an avocado, sprinkle it with a little sea salt, and enjoy. Avocados also pair well with a squeeze of lime and a sprinkle of chili flakes for an added flavor kick.

Greek yogurt, particularly the full-fat variety, is another excellent source of healthy fats. It provides beneficial probiotics for gut health along with protein and fat to keep you full. You can top it with a handful of seeds, a drizzle of honey, or some fresh fruit for added nutrition and flavor. If you're pressed for time, pre-packaged, individual servings of full-fat Greek yogurt can be a convenient on-the-go snack.

For those who enjoy a savory snack, roasted chickpeas or olives are perfect options. Both are rich in healthy fats and fiber, helping to satisfy cravings without adding excessive calories. Including healthy fat-rich snacks in your daily routine not only supports overall health but also helps stabilize blood sugar levels, preventing energy crashes.

## 3.3 Avoiding Hidden Fats

While it's important to include healthy fats in your diet, it's equally crucial to be aware of hidden fats that may be lurking in processed foods and takeout options. These hidden fats are often unhealthy and can negatively impact your health if consumed in excess. Being vigilant and reading food labels is key to avoiding these hidden sources of fat.

One of the most significant culprits of hidden fats is processed and packaged foods. Many snack foods, such as chips, cookies, and baked goods, contain trans fats, which are artificially created fats known to raise bad cholesterol (LDL) and increase the risk of heart disease. Even if a product claims to be "low fat," it may still contain unhealthy fats in the form of partially hydrogenated oils, which contribute to the presence of trans fats. Avoiding these foods and opting for whole, unprocessed alternatives will help you stay on track with your fat intake.

Restaurant and fast food meals can also be packed with hidden fats. Many sauces, dressings, and fried items are cooked in oils high in trans fats or unhealthy saturated fats. When dining out, request dressings and sauces on the side, and choose grilled or baked options over fried dishes to minimize your intake of unhealthy fats. Be mindful of the oils used for cooking and inquire about healthier alternatives if possible.

Additionally, packaged salad dressings, pre-made dips, and condiments like mayonnaise often contain unhealthy fats. Instead, make your own dressings at home using olive oil, lemon, and herbs, or opt for avocado as a creamy alternative. Even seemingly healthy foods, like granola bars or energy bars, can sometimes contain hidden fats in the form of added oils, so always check the ingredient list to ensure you're choosing whole food-based options.

By being proactive and avoiding hidden fats, you can ensure that your fat intake remains balanced and healthy. Focusing on whole, nutrient-dense foods and minimizing processed items is key to maintaining a diet rich in beneficial fats while steering clear of harmful alternatives.

Incorporating these practical fat tips into your daily routine can help you make the most of healthy fats, ensuring they enhance both the flavor and nutritional value of your meals. Whether you're cooking, snacking, or making more mindful choices about hidden fats, these strategies will empower you to build a well-rounded, sustainable diet that supports long-term health.

# Meal Timing and Frequency

## Why Timing Matters

### 1.1 The Role of Pre- and Post-Workout Nutrition

When it comes to maximizing performance and achieving your fitness goals, meal timing plays a pivotal role. Specifically, pre- and post-workout nutrition is essential to fueling your body for peak performance and optimizing recovery. What you eat, and when, can impact both your energy levels during the workout and the recovery process that follows.

Before you hit the gym, your body requires fuel. Pre-workout nutrition should focus on providing quick-digesting carbohydrates and moderate protein to replenish glycogen stores and supply your muscles with the necessary amino acids for protein synthesis. Consuming a balanced meal about 1 to 2 hours before your workout gives your body time to digest and absorb nutrients, ensuring your muscles are primed and ready. If you're short on time, a small snack, such as a banana or a protein shake, can be consumed 30 minutes prior to exercise. This approach helps improve performance by offering a steady stream of energy without causing discomfort during your workout.

Post-workout, your muscles are in a state of recovery, and this is where proper nutrition becomes even more crucial. Within 30 to 60 minutes after exercise, your body is most receptive to nutrients. During this "anabolic window," a combination of high-quality protein and fast-digesting carbohydrates helps replenish depleted glycogen stores, repair muscle tissue, and stimulate muscle growth. A post-workout meal, like a protein shake with a serving of fruit or a lean chicken and sweet potato combination, can accelerate recovery, reduce muscle soreness, and enhance your results.

The key to success with pre- and post-workout nutrition is timing. Failing to fuel properly before a workout can lead to fatigue and hinder performance, while neglecting post-workout nutrition can slow down recovery and muscle repair. To optimize energy, recovery, and results, prioritize the timing of your meals around your workouts and watch your performance and progress soar.

## 1.2 Timing Macros for Maximum Energy

To maintain consistent energy throughout the day, understanding how to time your macronutrients—proteins, fats, and carbohydrates—is critical. Your body needs a balance of these macros at strategic times to fuel energy, prevent muscle breakdown, and maintain overall health.

Carbohydrates are your body's primary source of energy, especially when you're engaging in high-intensity workouts or physical activity. However, the timing of carb consumption is just as important as the amount. Eating simple carbohydrates (e.g., fruits or white rice) right before a workout gives your muscles the quick energy boost they need, while complex carbohydrates (e.g., oatmeal or whole grains) provide sustained energy over a longer period and are best consumed during meals throughout the day.

Protein, on the other hand, is essential for muscle repair and growth. Consuming protein throughout the day, particularly in the form of high-quality sources such as lean meats, eggs, or plant-based alternatives, helps maintain a constant supply of amino acids in the bloodstream. Timing protein intake after workouts or spreading it out over multiple meals ensures your muscles are continuously supported. A common recommendation is to consume 20–30 grams of protein per meal, especially if you're trying to build muscle mass or improve recovery.

Fats are often overlooked when it comes to meal timing, but they too play an important role in maintaining energy and promoting overall health. Healthy fats, like those found in avocados, nuts, and olive oil, provide sustained energy and help absorb fat-soluble vitamins. However, consuming large amounts of fats immediately before or during a workout might slow digestion and cause discomfort. It's best to incorporate fats into meals that occur at least 2–3 hours before exercise.

By timing your macronutrient intake throughout the day—carbs for energy, protein for muscle repair, and fats for sustained energy—you can maximize your body's potential to perform at its best and recover more effectively.

## 1.3 Managing Hunger with Timing

One of the greatest challenges many face when pursuing fitness goals is managing hunger. You might feel the urge to snack constantly, especially if you're eating less to lose weight or adjusting your diet to build lean muscle. Interestingly, meal timing can help control hunger, reduce cravings, and even enhance weight management.

One effective way to curb hunger is by spreading meals out over the day, maintaining regular intervals of 3 to 4 hours between meals. This helps keep blood sugar levels stable, preventing spikes and crashes that can lead to intense hunger. Skipping meals or waiting too long between eating can trigger extreme hunger and lead to overeating later on. By consuming balanced meals at consistent times, you can better regulate appetite and avoid the temptation to snack excessively.

Incorporating protein into every meal is another key to managing hunger. Protein is known for its ability to promote feelings of fullness, and it has a higher thermic effect than carbohydrates and fats, meaning your body burns more calories digesting it. Eating a protein-rich breakfast, followed by protein at lunch and dinner, will help keep your appetite in check throughout the day. For example, a meal of grilled chicken, quinoa, and veggies offers protein, fiber, and healthy fats that will keep you satisfied.

Finally, be mindful of your carb timing as well. Consuming most of your carbohydrates earlier in the day, when your activity level is higher, can prevent sluggishness and excessive hunger in the evening. Simple, quick-digesting carbs, such as fruits or smoothies, make great mid-day snacks, offering a fast energy boost and reducing cravings for heavier, calorie-dense foods.

By strategically timing meals and focusing on protein and balanced macronutrients, you can maintain control over your hunger levels, which in turn supports your fitness goals, whether you're aiming to lose fat, build muscle, or maintain a healthy weight.

Through these key strategies—pre- and post-workout nutrition, optimized macro timing, and hunger management—meal timing becomes an essential tool in building your best body. It's not just about what you eat, but when you eat it, that can make all the difference in your energy levels, recovery, and long-term fitness success.

## Finding the Right Frequency

## 2.1 Meal Frequency: Fewer vs. More Meals

When it comes to meal frequency, there's no one-size-fits-all approach. Some people thrive on eating multiple smaller meals throughout the day, while others prefer fewer, larger meals. The key to finding the right frequency lies in understanding your personal goals, preferences, and lifestyle.

The traditional approach of eating three square meals a day has worked for many for generations. This structure allows the body to process meals with ample time between them, creating a feeling of fullness after each meal. However, there are benefits to eating more frequently, typically 4 to 6 meals per day. By doing so, you may be able to keep your metabolism more active, sustain energy levels throughout the day, and manage hunger better. Frequent meals, especially ones that include balanced amounts of protein, carbs, and fats, can help stabilize blood sugar and curb unhealthy cravings.

On the other hand, some individuals prefer eating fewer meals a day, such as 2 or 3 meals with larger portions. This approach can be equally effective for those who prefer fewer distractions throughout the day, or for those who find that eating larger meals satisfies them for longer periods of time. Fewer meals can also make it easier to control portion sizes, which is particularly beneficial for those looking to reduce calorie intake for fat loss. The reduced meal frequency may also improve digestion by allowing the body to focus more on the absorption and breakdown of food in longer intervals.

It's also worth considering that meal frequency can have an impact on muscle mass and fat loss. Eating more frequently allows for a steady stream of nutrients to the muscles, which is advantageous for individuals aiming to build muscle. Meanwhile, fewer meals may be effective for those looking to manage their weight and are comfortable with a more condensed eating window. Ultimately, the decision to eat more or fewer meals should be based on your personal goals—whether it's fat loss, muscle gain, or maintaining overall health—and what best suits your lifestyle.

## 2.2 Adapting Frequency to Your Schedule

One of the most important factors in meal frequency is how well it fits into your daily schedule. The key is to create a meal plan that is both sustainable and convenient, tailored to your daily life. For those with busy schedules, meal timing can sometimes be more about practicality than ideal macro distribution.

If you have a packed workday or a hectic lifestyle, the thought of preparing and eating multiple meals throughout the day may seem overwhelming. In this case, you can adapt your meal frequency by preparing your meals ahead of time or focusing on meal timing that fits within the natural gaps of your schedule. For example, if you're working long hours, having two main meals with a couple of healthy snacks in between can work wonders. Prepping meals in advance, such as overnight oats or meal prep bowls, ensures that you stay on track even during busy times, preventing poor food choices and allowing you to stick to your nutrition goals.

If you're someone who exercises in the morning, you might prefer to have your first meal post-workout, followed by lunch and dinner. This structure is simple and allows you to consume enough protein and calories for muscle recovery without overcomplicating things. Conversely, if you prefer evening workouts, you may want to focus on having a balanced meal before exercise and a substantial post-workout meal to fuel recovery overnight.

Personalizing meal frequency also means adjusting meal sizes. For some, having 3 larger meals with moderate snacks is more satisfying, while others might prefer 5 or 6 smaller meals spread throughout the day. If you're looking to manage hunger or avoid the mid-afternoon slump, more frequent meals can help keep energy levels high. Regardless of your schedule, the best approach is one that is consistent and that fits seamlessly into your daily life, making it easy to maintain over the long term.

## 2.3 The Role of Intermittent Fasting

Intermittent fasting (IF) has become an increasingly popular approach for those looking to manage their weight, optimize fat loss, or improve metabolic health. The principle of intermittent fasting revolves around alternating periods of eating and fasting, typically by following an eating window of 6 to 8 hours, while fasting for the remaining 16 to 18 hours of the day. But how does intermittent fasting align with your macros, and can it help you achieve your fitness goals?

When following an intermittent fasting regimen, the timing of macronutrient intake becomes critical. During the eating window, it's important to focus on consuming nutrient-dense, balanced meals that include the right amount of protein, carbs, and fats to fuel the body's energy needs. Protein becomes especially important during IF, as fasting periods can lead to muscle breakdown if your protein intake isn't sufficient. Including high-quality protein sources such as lean meats, fish, eggs, or plant-based protein ensures that your body has the necessary building blocks for muscle repair and growth. Consuming protein within your eating window is key to preserving muscle mass while you're in a caloric deficit for fat loss.

Carbohydrates also play a role during IF. Since you're eating fewer meals, the amount of carbs you consume during each meal should be well-calculated to ensure that your body has the necessary energy for activity and recovery. Carbs, especially complex ones like oats, quinoa, and sweet potatoes, provide sustained energy, helping you perform your best in the gym while keeping blood sugar levels stable throughout the fasting window.

Fats, which are slower to digest, are a great source of long-lasting energy during fasting hours. By incorporating healthy fats, such as those from nuts, seeds, avocado, and olive oil, you can help curb hunger and maintain satiety during the fasting period. These fats also support essential bodily functions, including hormone regulation, which is crucial for those focused on building muscle or maintaining overall health.

Incorporating intermittent fasting with the right macronutrient balance can be an effective strategy for weight loss, muscle preservation, and overall health. By focusing on what you eat and when you eat it, you can optimize the benefits of fasting while ensuring that your body is properly nourished to perform and recover optimally.

Meal frequency is about finding what works best for your lifestyle and goals. Whether you prefer fewer, larger meals or more frequent smaller ones, the key is consistency and personalization. Intermittent fasting can be an effective strategy for those looking to optimize fat loss or manage weight, as long as the right balance of macros is maintained within the eating window. By understanding your body's needs and adapting meal timing to your unique schedule, you can find the right frequency that supports your fitness journey.

# Practical Meal Timing

## 3.1 Scheduling Your Meals

Finding the time to eat healthy meals in a busy lifestyle can be challenging, but with some planning and organization, it's possible to stay on track with your nutrition goals. Scheduling your meals strategically is key to maintaining energy levels, boosting productivity, and supporting fitness results. Here are some practical strategies for fitting meals around your packed schedule.

First, assess your daily routine and identify natural windows for eating. If you have a job or other commitments that demand a lot of your time, try to find small pockets in your day where meals can be conveniently consumed. For example, if you have a long commute, you might use this time to enjoy a pre-packed breakfast or snack. If you're working at a desk or in meetings most of the day, try planning meals at specific times—perhaps a lunch break around midday and a snack in the late afternoon to keep your energy steady.

Meal prep is your best friend in this scenario. Preparing meals ahead of time allows you to avoid scrambling for something healthy when you're hungry and pressed for time. Consider dedicating a few hours each weekend to cook in bulk, portioning out meals for the week. Foods like grilled chicken, quinoa, roasted vegetables, and hard-boiled eggs are easy to prepare in advance and store in the fridge. Batch cooking not only saves time during the week but also ensures that you're eating the right macronutrients without the temptation to opt for less nutritious, time-saving alternatives.

If you find it difficult to sit down for a full meal during busy hours, consider smaller, portable meals or snacks. Protein shakes, protein bars, or pre-packaged salads are excellent options for those on the go, providing necessary nutrients without requiring a lot of time or preparation. These portable options ensure you still have the energy to perform your daily tasks and stay on track with your nutrition goals.

## 3.2 Balancing Work, Life, and Nutrition

Balancing work, life, and nutrition can seem overwhelming, but with the right tools and strategies, it's entirely achievable. One of the most effective ways to ensure consistency is through meal prep and planning. By taking the time to prepare your meals in advance, you can avoid the stress of last-minute decisions and make it easier to stick to your nutrition goals.

Meal prepping doesn't have to mean spending hours in the kitchen. A simple and efficient strategy is to batch-cook the basics—proteins, grains, and vegetables—and mix and match them throughout the week. For example, cook a large portion of chicken, brown rice, and roasted veggies on Sunday, and divide them into portions that can be easily grabbed and reheated for lunch or dinner. This method provides flexibility while ensuring you have nutrient-dense meals readily available, saving you time and reducing the temptation to grab unhealthy options.

Another strategy is to keep your kitchen stocked with healthy ingredients that can be easily assembled. Think of it as a "meal assembly line." For example, having pre-washed leafy greens, canned tuna or beans, and whole-grain wraps on hand allows you to quickly throw together a salad or wrap when you don't have time for cooking. These meals don't require a lot of preparation, but they still provide the necessary nutrients to keep you energized throughout the day.

A good way to balance work and life with nutrition is to prioritize consistency over perfection. It's about creating habits that allow you to maintain your nutrition goals despite the chaos of everyday life. Whether it's having a meal plan that you follow for a few days or investing in a meal delivery service, consistency in meal timing and preparation is more important than striving for a perfect, rigid routine.

## 3.3 Tips for Staying Consistent

Consistency is the cornerstone of long-term success in both nutrition and fitness. Staying consistent with meal timing requires creating habits that are manageable, sustainable, and adaptable to your lifestyle. Here are some tips to help you stay on track:

**1. Plan Ahead**: The key to consistency is preparation. Set aside time each week to plan your meals, make a grocery list, and prep your food. Knowing exactly what you're going to eat helps eliminate decision fatigue and reduces the temptation to make poor food choices.

**2. Build a Routine**: Establishing a meal routine can make eating well a habit, not a task. Eat at regular intervals and aim to consume meals at similar times each day. Consistency in meal timing helps regulate your metabolism and keeps hunger at bay, reducing the likelihood of overeating or making unhealthy food choices when you're too hungry.

**3. Batch Cook and Store**: Dedicate time to cook in bulk, and store meals in containers for the week. This simple habit can save you time and stress throughout the week, allowing you to stay consistent even when you're short on time. When you have meals prepped and ready to go, there's no excuse to skip or rush meals.

**4. Don't Skip Meals**: Skipping meals can lead to overeating later in the day and disrupt your blood sugar levels, which can affect your energy and mood. It's important to prioritize regular meals and snacks that contain the right balance of macronutrients to keep you feeling satisfied and energized.

**5. Be Flexible**: Life happens. There will be days when your meal timing doesn't go according to plan, and that's okay. The key is to not let one off day derail your progress. Adapt to your circumstances and adjust when necessary, but don't use it as an excuse to abandon your overall goals. Flexibility is a part of consistency.

**6. Track Progress**: Keep track of how meal timing impacts your energy, workouts, and hunger levels. Monitoring your progress can provide valuable insight into what works best for your body and help you make adjustments as needed. Whether through a food diary or an app, tracking allows you to stay accountable and motivated.

Ultimately, consistency isn't about being perfect every day. It's about creating a rhythm that supports your goals and sticking to it over time. By building a routine, planning ahead, and being flexible when necessary, you'll develop the habits that lead to long-term success in both nutrition and fitness.

If you may know, practical meal timing involves not just planning your meals, but creating a lifestyle that supports consistent, sustainable habits. Whether you're managing a busy career or personal commitments, scheduling meals around your day, balancing work-life with meal prep, and cultivating habits that encourage consistency will help you stay on track. The effort you put into planning, preparing, and sticking to your meals will pay off in your energy levels, fitness results, and long-term success.

# Macro Adjustments for Fat Loss

## Creating a Caloric Deficit

### 1.1 How a Deficit Leads to Fat Loss

Understanding the science behind fat loss is key to achieving sustainable results. Fat loss fundamentally revolves around creating a caloric deficit, a state where your body consumes fewer calories than it expends. This prompts your body to tap into stored energy, primarily from fat reserves, to meet its energy demands.

Every calorie you consume serves as fuel for essential bodily functions like breathing, digestion, and physical activity. When you consistently eat more calories than your body burns, the excess energy is stored as fat, leading to weight gain. Conversely, consuming fewer calories than your body requires triggers it to utilize fat stores to make up the shortfall. This process underpins fat loss.

However, achieving a caloric deficit isn't just about eating less—it's about balancing intake and expenditure effectively. Your basal metabolic rate (BMR), which is the energy your body needs to function at rest, accounts for the majority of your daily caloric burn. Adding physical activity and considering the thermic effect of food—calories burned through digestion—creates a dynamic interplay of energy balance.

The size of the deficit matters significantly. A moderate caloric deficit of about 500 calories per day is a practical target for most people, translating to a sustainable fat loss rate of approximately one pound per week. This approach minimizes the risks of muscle loss and metabolic slowdown, ensuring that your weight loss is both healthy and maintainable.

As you explore strategies to create this deficit, remember that this is only the foundation of your fat loss journey. The key to long-term success lies in the methods you adopt to make this adjustment sustainable, a topic we'll explore in the next section.

## 1.2 Avoiding Drastic Cuts

While it's tempting to drastically slash calories for quick results, this approach often leads to burnout and potential health risks. Instead, sustainable fat loss thrives on moderate reductions that allow for consistency and adaptability.

Severe calorie cuts can trigger your body's natural defense: metabolic adaptation. This slows down your metabolism, making it harder to lose weight over time. Moreover, drastic reductions can lead to muscle loss, energy depletion, and nutritional deficiencies that compromise your overall well-being. Psychologically, they can foster feelings of deprivation, increasing the likelihood of binge eating or abandoning your goals altogether.

Moderation is key. A deficit of around 500 calories per day is both effective and manageable for most people. This not only supports gradual fat loss but also preserves lean muscle mass and keeps your metabolism active. Pairing this approach with nutrient-dense foods—like lean proteins, whole grains, fruits, and vegetables—ensures that you're fueling your body with essential nutrients while staying within your caloric limit.

Equally important is the distribution of calories throughout your day. Spacing meals and snacks evenly helps maintain steady blood sugar levels, preventing energy crashes and excessive hunger. This promotes adherence to your plan without the frustration of constant cravings.

By adopting this sustainable approach, you're laying the groundwork for long-term success. But fat loss isn't just about cutting calories; it's about finding a balance that keeps your energy levels high while staying committed to your goals. This balance is the focus of the next section.

## 1.3 Balancing Fat Loss and Energy

Sustaining energy while in a caloric deficit is a delicate balancing act, yet it's essential for ensuring both progress and vitality. To effectively balance fat loss and energy, your approach should prioritize quality nutrition, strategic meal planning, and physical activity that enhances your metabolic health.

Nutrient-dense foods are your best allies. Lean proteins help preserve muscle mass and promote satiety, while whole grains provide a steady source of energy. Including healthy fats and fiber-rich vegetables ensures your meals are balanced and satisfying. Together, these foods not only keep you energized but also help you stick to your caloric target without feeling deprived.

Meal timing also plays a crucial role. Eating smaller, frequent meals throughout the day can stabilize blood sugar levels and prevent the dips in energy that often accompany extended periods of hunger. Incorporating snacks with protein and complex carbohydrates—like a handful of nuts or Greek yogurt with fruit—can help you maintain focus and productivity.

Physical activity further complements this balance. Cardiovascular exercises increase caloric burn, while strength training preserves muscle mass, keeping your metabolism active. Prioritizing movement also contributes to a stronger, healthier body that's better equipped to handle the demands of fat loss.

As you adjust to these strategies, remain attuned to your body's signals. Fatigue, irritability, or persistent hunger may indicate that your deficit is too aggressive, warranting a reassessment. The journey to fat loss isn't linear, but with careful adjustments, you'll find a rhythm that works for you.

This interplay between nutrition, energy, and activity creates a harmonious cycle—one that not only supports fat loss but also builds the foundation for a healthier, more sustainable lifestyle.

# Monitoring Progress

## 2.1 Signs Your Plan is Working

Monitoring progress effectively is crucial for staying motivated and ensuring that your fat loss plan is on the right track. While the scale often becomes the default measure, there are other, more insightful indicators that reveal whether your efforts are paying off.

The first sign of success is changes in how your clothes fit. A looser waistband or a more comfortable fit in your favorite outfit often signals fat loss, even if the number on the scale isn't moving as expected. This occurs because your body composition—how much of you is muscle versus fat—can change even when your weight remains stable.

Improved energy levels and better mood are also positive indicators. As you fine-tune your macros and incorporate nutrient-dense foods, your body benefits from more stable blood sugar levels and improved digestion. These changes manifest in fewer energy crashes, increased productivity, and enhanced focus.

Another key sign is progress in your workouts. Increased strength, better endurance, or improved recovery times indicate that your body is adapting to your fitness regimen while preserving or building muscle mass. This is a clear sign that your approach is supporting a healthy metabolism and effective fat loss.

Lastly, look for reductions in body measurements, such as waist or hip circumference. Tracking these regularly provides a more accurate picture of fat loss than relying solely on weight, as muscle gain or water retention can obscure scale results.

These early successes are important milestones, but they're only the beginning. To ensure continued progress, it's essential to measure your results accurately and make informed adjustments. This leads us to the next section.

## 2.2 Tracking Fat Loss Accurately

Accurate tracking is the cornerstone of effective fat loss. Without reliable data, it's easy to misjudge progress and make unnecessary or counterproductive changes. By using a combination of methods, you can gain a clearer picture of your journey.

One of the simplest ways to track fat loss is by measuring body weight. However, weight fluctuations due to water retention, hormonal changes, or digestion can distort short-term results. To mitigate this, weigh yourself at the same time every morning, ideally after using the bathroom and before eating or drinking. Use weekly averages rather than daily readings to assess trends over time.

Body measurements, such as waist, hips, chest, and thighs, provide a more detailed perspective on fat loss. These measurements capture changes in body composition that the scale might miss, especially if you're gaining muscle while losing fat.

Progress photos are another invaluable tool. Taking photos from consistent angles under similar lighting conditions can reveal subtle changes in your physique. Reviewing these images over time often highlights progress that isn't immediately visible in the mirror.

For a more precise assessment, consider tools like body fat calipers, bioelectrical impedance devices, or professional services like DEXA scans. These methods estimate body fat percentage, offering deeper insights into changes in body composition.

Finally, maintain a food and activity log to correlate your dietary habits and exercise with your results. Apps or journals help you identify patterns, ensuring you stay accountable to your plan.

Tracking isn't about perfection but about understanding trends and making informed decisions. When progress slows or stalls, it's time to examine the data and adjust your approach—a topic we'll cover next.

## 2.3 Adjusting Macros to Break Plateaus

Even the most carefully designed plans can hit a plateau. When progress stalls, refining your macronutrient ratios is often the key to reigniting fat loss. Plateaus occur because your body adapts to its environment, including reduced caloric intake or increased activity. To overcome this, strategic adjustments are necessary.

The first step is to revisit your current caloric intake. As you lose weight, your caloric needs decrease because a smaller body requires less energy to maintain. Recalculate your caloric needs based on your new weight and activity level, then adjust your macros to maintain the desired deficit.

Start with protein, which should remain consistent or even increase during plateaus to preserve muscle mass. Aim for 0.8 to 1.2 grams of protein per pound of body weight. Next, evaluate your fat and carbohydrate intake. Reducing fats slightly or cycling carbohydrates around workout days can provide the caloric reduction needed to break the plateau without compromising energy levels.

Another strategy involves introducing refeed days, where you temporarily increase caloric intake, primarily through carbohydrates. Refeeds can boost leptin levels, a hormone that regulates hunger and metabolism, helping to counteract the metabolic slowdown often associated with prolonged deficits.

Additionally, assess your physical activity. If your current routine has become less challenging, incorporating higher-intensity workouts or increasing training volume can help stimulate further fat loss. Non-exercise activity thermogenesis (NEAT), like walking or fidgeting, can also play a role in boosting your overall energy expenditure.

Breaking plateaus requires patience and careful experimentation. Regularly track your adjustments and monitor their effects to ensure that your changes are effective and sustainable. This iterative process will keep your fat loss journey progressing and set the stage for long-term success.

# Long-Term Fat Loss

## 3.1 Maintaining Muscle While Losing Fat

Preserving muscle mass is not just a bonus during fat loss—it's a necessity for achieving a strong, lean, and healthy body. Losing fat while maintaining muscle ensures you retain your metabolic efficiency, strength, and overall vitality, even as the scale moves down.

To achieve this, nutrition plays a central role. Protein is the cornerstone of muscle preservation, providing your body with the essential amino acids it needs to repair and rebuild muscle tissue. Aim for 0.8 to 1.2 grams of protein per pound of body weight daily, spacing this intake evenly across meals to optimize muscle protein synthesis.

Equally important is your training regimen. Resistance exercises signal your body to hold onto muscle by emphasizing strength and performance. Focus on compound movements like squats, deadlifts, and presses, and aim for at least 2–4 strength training sessions per week. The goal isn't to work harder but smarter, adjusting intensity and volume to match your energy levels during a caloric deficit.

Gradual weight loss is another critical factor. Rapid fat loss often triggers muscle breakdown, leaving your metabolism weaker and less efficient. Aim for a steady loss of 0.5–1% of your body weight per week to ensure you're primarily shedding fat, not muscle.

Finally, prioritize recovery through quality sleep and stress management. Sleep regulates the hormones that control muscle repair and fat metabolism, while managing stress helps minimize cortisol, which can contribute to muscle loss.

Maintaining muscle while losing fat sets the foundation for long-term success. But muscle retention alone isn't enough—your approach must also be sustainable. Let's explore how to make gradual adjustments that you can stick with over time.

## 3.2 Sustainable Caloric Adjustments

Fat loss that lasts requires changes you can live with, not short-term fixes. Sustainable caloric adjustments help you stay consistent while avoiding the common pitfalls of crash diets and extreme measures.

Start by understanding your maintenance calories—the number of calories you need to maintain your current weight. From there, create a modest deficit of 10–20%, which is small enough to avoid feelings of deprivation while still driving fat loss. This gradual approach allows your body to adapt over time, reducing the risk of burnout or metabolic slowdown.

As your weight decreases, your caloric needs will change. Periodically reassess your intake every 4–6 weeks, making minor adjustments if progress slows. This ensures your deficit remains effective without drastic cuts that can sap your energy or harm your progress.

Flexibility is key to sustainability. Instead of eliminating entire food groups, focus on balance within your macros. For example, enjoy nutrient-dense meals most of the time but allow for occasional indulgences. This flexible approach helps you maintain a positive relationship with food, reducing the likelihood of feeling restricted or giving up altogether.

Practical habits also make sustainability easier. Meal prepping, tracking your intake, and prioritizing whole foods simplify decision-making, keeping you on track even during busy days. Consistency, not perfection, is what drives long-term success.

By adopting manageable changes, you're building a plan that supports not just fat loss but a healthy lifestyle. But even with a solid strategy, staying motivated is essential to keep progressing—our focus in the next section.

## 3.3 Staying Motivated

Long-term fat loss isn't just about the physical changes—it's a mental journey, too. Staying motivated requires reconnecting with your goals, building habits that support your lifestyle, and navigating challenges with resilience.

Start by defining a clear and meaningful "why." Whether it's improving your health, boosting confidence, or achieving specific fitness milestones, your purpose will act as a compass when motivation wanes. Write it down, visualize the outcome, and remind yourself regularly of what you're working toward.

Set realistic, measurable goals and break them into smaller milestones. Achieving a goal like losing 5 pounds or completing a new fitness challenge builds momentum and reinforces your commitment. Celebrate each win—it's a reminder of your progress and potential.

Habits are the backbone of sustained motivation. Incorporate consistent practices, like scheduling workouts, prepping meals, or setting aside time for mindfulness. Over time, these behaviors become automatic, reducing the mental energy needed to stay on track.

When plateaus or setbacks arise, view them as opportunities to reassess and adapt. Reflect on what's working, and seek support when needed. Join fitness communities, work with a coach, or share your journey with friends and family. These connections foster accountability and encouragement, helping you stay focused even during tough times.

Finally, keep things fresh by introducing variety. Experiment with new workouts, try different recipes, or set creative fitness challenges. Variety keeps your routine exciting, reducing the risk of boredom or burnout.

Motivation ebbs and flows, but by building a system of habits, support, and personal meaning, you can sustain your efforts for the long haul. With a clear vision and a flexible approach, long-term fat loss becomes not just achievable but a natural part of your healthier lifestyle.

# Macro Adjustments for Muscle Gain

## Understanding a Caloric Surplus

### 1.1 Why Muscle Growth Requires Extra Calories

Muscle growth, also known as hypertrophy, is an energy-intensive process that begins with resistance training. When you lift weights or perform other strength-building exercises, your muscles experience micro-tears. To repair these fibers and make them stronger and larger, your body needs a steady supply of energy, which comes from the calories you consume. This is why simply eating at maintenance—where calorie intake equals calorie expenditure—is insufficient for optimal muscle growth.

A caloric surplus provides the additional fuel necessary for repair and growth. Think of it as giving your body the raw materials it needs to build something new. Without these extra calories, your body might struggle to repair damaged tissue, potentially compromising your results and even burning muscle during prolonged deficits.

However, not all calories are created equal. A surplus built on nutrient-dense foods—such as lean proteins, whole grains, and healthy fats—ensures your muscles receive the building blocks they need, like amino acids for protein synthesis and glycogen to replenish energy stores. Research suggests a surplus of 10–20% above maintenance is optimal for gradual, quality muscle growth. For example, if your maintenance calories are 2,500 per day, consuming 2,750–3,000 calories creates a productive environment for gains.

By understanding the need for a caloric surplus and focusing on quality nutrition, you can effectively support your body's muscle-building processes while minimizing the risk of unwanted fat gain.

## 1.2 How to Avoid Overeating

While a caloric surplus is necessary for muscle gain, consuming too many calories can lead to excessive fat accumulation. Striking the right balance is crucial, and it begins with accurately determining your daily caloric needs. Once you've established your maintenance level, adding a modest 250–500 calories ensures you're in a surplus without going overboard.

To prevent overeating, pay attention to portion sizes and meal timing. Spreading your caloric intake over 4–6 meals per day can help maintain energy levels and avoid overwhelming hunger that might lead to binge eating. Tracking your food intake using apps or journals also provides clarity on whether you're staying within your surplus target.

Another strategy involves mindful eating. Slowing down during meals and tuning into your body's hunger cues can prevent you from consuming more than necessary. Remember, eating for muscle growth isn't about stuffing yourself but about making every calorie count.

Resistance training can also act as a safeguard against minor overconsumption. The extra energy you consume is often channeled toward muscle repair and glycogen replenishment rather than fat storage. With these strategies in place, you can strike the perfect balance, ensuring your surplus serves its purpose effectively.

## 1.3 The Slow and Steady Approach

Building muscle is a marathon, not a sprint. While it's tempting to aim for rapid weight gain, this approach often results in excessive fat accumulation alongside muscle growth. Instead, a gradual pace—aiming to gain 0.25–0.5% of your body weight per week—allows for sustainable and primarily lean mass increases.

This slow approach is not only healthier but also gives your body time to adapt. Rapid changes in weight can lead to metabolic inefficiencies, making it harder to maintain lean muscle over the long term. For example, if you weigh 160 pounds, targeting 0.4–0.8 pounds per week ensures your progress is controlled and primarily muscle-driven.

Tracking your progress through body measurements and performance metrics can help you stay on course. If your lifts are improving, your energy is high, and your body composition remains favorable, you're likely in the sweet spot for growth. Adjust your

# Fine-Tuning Macros for Growth

## 2.1 Protein for Muscle Building

Protein is the cornerstone of muscle growth. When you engage in resistance training, your muscles undergo stress, leading to microscopic tears in the fibers. Protein provides the amino acids your body needs to repair and rebuild these fibers, making them stronger and larger. This process, known as protein synthesis, is vital for hypertrophy and overall muscle health.

To optimize muscle growth, consuming an adequate amount of protein daily is non-negotiable. Experts recommend aiming for 1.6–2.2 grams of protein per kilogram of body weight. For instance, if you weigh 70 kilograms (154 pounds), your target protein intake should range between 112 and 154 grams per day. This ensures your body has a steady supply of the building blocks needed to support muscle repair.

Timing also plays a role in protein utilization. Consuming protein-rich meals evenly spaced throughout the day—especially within the anabolic window (30–60 minutes post-workout)—can maximize protein synthesis. Foods like chicken, fish, eggs, tofu, and dairy products are excellent protein sources, providing a mix of essential amino acids.

Supplementing with protein powders, such as whey or casein, can also help meet your daily targets, especially for individuals with high protein requirements or busy schedules. By prioritizing protein intake and focusing on quality sources, you set the stage for effective muscle repair and long-term growth.

## 2.2 Carbs for Recovery and Energy

While protein often takes center stage in muscle-building discussions, carbohydrates are equally critical. Carbs serve as your body's primary energy source, fueling workouts and aiding recovery post-exercise. When you train intensely, your glycogen stores—carbs stored in your muscles—are depleted. Replenishing these stores is essential to prepare for your next session and ensure optimal performance.

Carbohydrates also play a role in muscle recovery. Consuming carbs alongside protein after a workout has been shown to enhance glycogen replenishment and support muscle repair. This combination stimulates insulin release, which helps shuttle nutrients like glucose and amino acids into muscle cells.

Aiming for 3–6 grams of carbohydrates per kilogram of body weight daily can support muscle growth and recovery. For example, a 70-kilogram individual should consume 210–420 grams of carbs daily, depending on activity level. Prioritize complex carbohydrates, such as oats, sweet potatoes, quinoa, and whole grains, which provide sustained energy. Simple carbs, like fruits or honey, can be beneficial immediately after workouts due to their rapid absorption.

Carbs are not just fuel; they are the spark that keeps your workouts intense and your muscles ready to grow. By making carbohydrates a cornerstone of your diet, you ensure sustained energy and effective recovery.

## 2.3 Fats for Hormonal Balance

Fats often get a bad rap, but they are indispensable for muscle growth. Healthy fats play a critical role in maintaining hormonal balance, particularly in supporting the production of anabolic hormones like testosterone. These hormones directly influence muscle repair, protein synthesis, and overall growth.

Incorporating 20–30% of your daily calories from fat is a good rule of thumb. For example, if your caloric target is 3,000 calories, 600–900 calories should come from fat, equating to 67–100 grams. Prioritize healthy fats from sources like avocados, nuts, seeds, olive oil, and fatty fish such as salmon or mackerel. These foods are rich in omega-3 and monounsaturated fats, which support heart health and reduce inflammation—both essential for recovery.

Saturated fats, found in foods like eggs and lean meats, also have their place, contributing to testosterone production. However, limit trans fats, commonly found in processed and fried foods, as they can negatively impact health and performance.

Fats also provide a concentrated source of energy, which can be particularly beneficial for individuals with high caloric needs during a muscle-building phase. By incorporating healthy fats into your diet, you not only support hormonal health but also ensure your body has the resources to sustain long-term growth.

# Tracking Progress

## 3.1 Measuring Muscle Growth

Tracking muscle growth is an essential component of any muscle-building journey. Without proper monitoring, it's easy to lose sight of your progress or misinterpret changes in your body composition. Accurate tracking ensures that your efforts in the gym and kitchen align with your goals.

One of the most reliable ways to measure muscle growth is through body composition analysis. Methods like bioelectrical impedance scales, DEXA scans, or caliper measurements provide insights into your lean mass versus fat mass. While these tools can vary in accuracy, using the same method consistently gives a clear trend over time.

Another practical approach is to track physical measurements. Regularly measuring key areas, such as your arms, chest, thighs, and waist, can highlight growth patterns. For example, if your arm circumference increases while your waist measurement remains steady, it's a good indicator of lean muscle gain. Pair these measurements with progress photos taken under similar lighting and angles for a visual record of your transformation.

Strength progression in the gym is another telltale sign of muscle growth. If your lifts are steadily improving—whether it's benching heavier weights or doing more reps—it's a strong indicator that your muscles are adapting and growing. Pair this with how you feel during workouts; increased stamina and performance are often tied to successful muscle building.

Lastly, consider using a journal or app to document your progress. By keeping track of your weight, body measurements, and workout performance, you can pinpoint trends and make adjustments as needed. Consistent tracking helps you stay accountable and ensures you're on the right path to building your best body.

## 3.2 Adjusting Macros as You Build Muscle

As you gain muscle, your body's caloric needs will change, and so should your macronutrient intake. This dynamic process ensures that your energy and nutrient levels remain optimized for continued growth.

Start by regularly reassessing your maintenance calories. As your muscle mass increases, your metabolism speeds up, requiring more energy to maintain and build new tissue. Adjust your calorie intake upward by 100–200 calories at a time to accommodate this growth.

Protein needs also evolve with your progress. While 1.6–2.2 grams per kilogram of body weight is a solid baseline, recalculating this as your weight changes ensures you meet your muscle repair and synthesis demands. Similarly, carbohydrate intake should scale with your activity level to maintain glycogen stores and fuel your workouts.

Fats remain critical for hormonal health, but their intake can stay proportionate to your total calories (20–30%). As your calorie intake rises, your fat intake will naturally increase in line with this percentage, ensuring consistent support for growth and recovery.

Tracking how your body responds to these changes is crucial. If you notice slowed progress, fatigue, or increased fat gain, it may signal the need for macro adjustments. Regularly evaluating your macros based on your goals and results ensures a steady trajectory toward muscle growth without unnecessary fat accumulation.

## 3.3 Avoiding Common Bulking Mistakes

Bulking can yield tremendous results when done correctly, but missteps can derail your progress. One common mistake is overeating, often under the guise of "bulking." While a caloric surplus is essential, consuming far beyond what your body needs leads to excessive fat gain, making future cutting phases more challenging.

To avoid this, maintain a modest surplus of 10–20% above your maintenance calories. Track your intake consistently and focus on nutrient-dense foods rather than relying on processed, calorie-dense options. Junk foods may quickly add calories, but they often lack the essential nutrients needed for muscle repair and performance.

Another pitfall is neglecting cardio. Many believe that cardio burns muscle, but moderate cardiovascular activity supports heart health, enhances recovery, and can help manage fat gain during bulking phases. Incorporating 2–3 low-impact sessions weekly can complement your muscle-building efforts without hindering progress.

Finally, impatience is a bulking enemy. Trying to rush muscle gain by drastically increasing calories or skipping proper tracking can lead to frustration. Remember, muscle building is a gradual process that rewards consistency over time.

By staying mindful of these potential missteps, you can navigate your bulking phase effectively, ensuring every effort aligns with building your best body.

# The Role of Hydration in Macro Nutrition

## Why Hydration Matte

### 1.1 How Water Supports Metabolism

Hydration is often overlooked in the context of nutrition, yet it plays a critical role in both fat loss and muscle gain. Water is the medium in which nearly all metabolic processes occur, making it essential for efficient nutrient utilization and energy production. Without adequate hydration, your body's ability to metabolize fats, synthesize proteins, and recover from workouts diminishes significantly.

For fat loss, water is integral to lipolysis, the process by which fat is broken down for energy. Studies have shown that even mild dehydration can slow down metabolic rates, making it harder for your body to burn calories effectively. Drinking enough water ensures that your metabolism operates at peak efficiency, supporting calorie burning throughout the day.

In muscle gain, water is equally important. Muscles are composed of approximately 75% water, and proper hydration enhances protein synthesis—the process responsible for muscle repair and growth. Additionally, water helps transport nutrients like amino acids, glucose, and electrolytes to muscle cells, ensuring they receive the fuel they need to recover and grow after intense workouts.

Beyond metabolic functions, staying hydrated supports digestion and absorption. Proper hydration ensures that your body can effectively break down macronutrients like proteins, fats, and carbohydrates into usable energy. This process not only fuels workouts but also aids recovery.

To optimize hydration for metabolism, aim to drink water consistently throughout the day rather than in large quantities at once. A good starting point is consuming half your body weight in ounces of water daily and adjusting based on activity level. By prioritizing water intake, you create a foundation for improved metabolic health, supporting your macro-nutrient goals.

## 1.2 The Impact of Dehydration on Performance

Dehydration can significantly impact your workout performance and overall fitness progress. Losing as little as 2% of your body weight in fluids can impair physical performance, leading to fatigue, reduced strength, and decreased endurance.

During exercise, your body loses water through sweat to regulate temperature. If this loss isn't replenished, dehydration sets in, disrupting muscle function and coordination. Dehydrated muscles are more prone to cramping, reducing your ability to perform at your best. Furthermore, insufficient hydration impairs the body's ability to deliver oxygen and nutrients to working muscles, hindering recovery and adaptation.

Cognitive function is also affected by dehydration, making it harder to maintain focus during workouts. This mental fatigue can lead to poor form, increasing the risk of injury. In strength training, dehydration reduces muscle contractions' efficiency, meaning you may lift less weight or complete fewer reps.

For athletes pursuing muscle gain, dehydration reduces cell volumization—a process where hydrated muscle cells signal the body to synthesize proteins. When hydration levels drop, this anabolic signal weakens, slowing muscle repair and growth. Similarly, those focusing on fat loss may find their workouts less effective, as dehydration can lower energy levels and make it harder to burn calories.

To prevent dehydration, monitor your sweat rate and adjust your water intake accordingly. Incorporating electrolytes like sodium and potassium can help maintain fluid balance, especially during prolonged or intense exercise. By staying hydrated, you protect your performance and maximize your results in the gym.

## 1.3 Staying Hydrated with Macros in Mind

Balancing hydration with macro-focused nutrition can seem challenging, but the two go hand in hand. Proper hydration not only supports your body's metabolic processes but also aids in the digestion and absorption of macronutrients, ensuring they work effectively toward your fitness goals.

Start by timing your water intake strategically around meals and workouts. Drinking water before meals can help regulate appetite, making it easier to stick to your macro targets without overeating. Sipping water during workouts replenishes fluids lost through sweat and supports energy delivery to your muscles.

Incorporating hydrating foods into your diet is another effective strategy. Foods like cucumbers, watermelon, and oranges are rich in water and also provide valuable vitamins and minerals. These foods complement a macro-balanced diet by adding hydration and micronutrients without excess calories.

For those tracking macros, be mindful of how beverages like protein shakes or flavored waters contribute to your daily intake. Opt for low-calorie, high-nutrient options that align with your macro goals while keeping you hydrated.

Electrolytes play a crucial role in hydration. When focusing on macros, it's important to maintain electrolyte balance to avoid water retention or dehydration. Adding a pinch of salt to your meals or using electrolyte supplements can help replenish sodium and potassium lost during workouts.

Finally, monitor your hydration levels by checking urine color—it should be pale yellow—and adjusting water intake as needed. Apps and smart water bottles can also remind you to drink regularly throughout the day. By integrating these strategies, you can maintain optimal hydration while keeping your macro goals on track, ensuring that both nutrition and hydration work together for peak performance.

# Best Hydration Practices

## 2.1 Water Intake Recommendations

Water is indispensable for overall health and performance, yet determining the right amount to drink daily can be confusing. While generalized guidelines suggest 8 cups (64 ounces) of water per day, hydration needs vary based on factors like body weight, activity level, and environmental conditions. For those pursuing fitness goals, proper water intake is critical to support muscle function, fat metabolism, and overall well-being.

A widely accepted approach for determining water needs is to consume half your body weight in ounces daily. For instance, a 160-pound individual should aim for approximately 80 ounces of water per day. However, athletes and active individuals often require more due to the increased water loss through sweat. On workout days, adding an extra 12–16 ounces for every 30 minutes of exercise is a good rule of thumb.

Thirst is a natural indicator of hydration needs, but it's not always reliable. By the time you feel thirsty, you may already be mildly dehydrated. Monitoring urine color is a more accurate way to assess hydration—pale yellow indicates adequate hydration, while dark yellow suggests you need to drink more water.

Staying consistent with water intake throughout the day is crucial. Instead of consuming large amounts all at once, sip water regularly. Using a water bottle with volume markers can help you track your intake and ensure you meet your daily goals. Apps and hydration trackers can also provide helpful reminders.

Hydrating properly doesn't mean relying solely on water. Herbal teas, sparkling water, and water-rich foods like fruits and vegetables contribute to your total intake. Foods such as cucumbers, oranges, and melons not only hydrate but also provide vitamins and minerals to support recovery and performance.

In summary, meeting your daily water needs is foundational for achieving fitness goals. By understanding your unique requirements and adopting consistent hydration habits, you create the conditions for optimal metabolic function, muscle performance, and overall health.

## 2.2 Electrolytes and Hydration

While water is essential for hydration, electrolytes are equally important in maintaining fluid balance and muscle function. Electrolytes—minerals like sodium, potassium, calcium, and magnesium—regulate water distribution in the body, support nerve signaling, and ensure proper muscle contractions. Without them, even adequate water intake may not prevent dehydration-related issues.

During exercise, sweat causes a loss of electrolytes, particularly sodium. If not replenished, this imbalance can lead to symptoms like muscle cramps, fatigue, and impaired performance. Sodium plays a key role in retaining water in the bloodstream, preventing excessive dehydration. Potassium complements sodium by helping muscles contract and relax efficiently, while magnesium and calcium support overall muscle function and energy production.

Electrolyte imbalances can occur even with a high water intake. For instance, overhydration without adequate sodium levels can cause a condition called hyponatremia, where sodium concentrations in the blood drop too low. This can result in dizziness, confusion, and even life-threatening complications.

To maintain optimal electrolyte balance, focus on nutrient-rich foods and, when necessary, supplements. Foods like bananas, leafy greens, nuts, and dairy are excellent sources of potassium, magnesium, and calcium. Adding a pinch of salt to meals or consuming sports drinks during intense workouts can help replenish sodium lost through sweat.

For endurance athletes or those training in hot conditions, consider electrolyte tablets or powders mixed with water. These provide a precise balance of minerals to sustain hydration and performance. However, be cautious of sugary sports drinks, which may contribute unnecessary calories and disrupt your macro goals.

Ultimately, balancing water and electrolyte intake ensures your body functions optimally during workouts and recovery. By addressing both hydration components, you can prevent cramps, sustain energy, and improve overall physical performance.

## 2.3 Hydration Strategies During Workouts

Maintaining proper hydration during workouts is vital for maximizing performance and recovery. Exercise increases sweat production, leading to water and electrolyte loss, which, if unchecked, can impair strength, endurance, and focus. Adopting effective hydration strategies ensures your body stays fueled and functional throughout your training sessions.

Begin your workout hydrated. Drink 12–16 ounces of water about 2 hours before exercise to ensure adequate fluid levels. Just before starting, consume another 8 ounces to top off your reserves. This pre-workout hydration minimizes the risk of starting dehydrated, which can negatively affect performance.

During exercise, aim to drink 4–8 ounces of water every 15–20 minutes, depending on sweat rate and workout intensity. If your session lasts under an hour, plain water is sufficient. For longer or more intense workouts, incorporate electrolyte-enhanced beverages to replenish lost sodium, potassium, and magnesium.

Temperature and workout conditions play a role in hydration needs. In hot and humid environments, your sweat rate increases, requiring more frequent hydration. Similarly, high-intensity exercises demand quicker replenishment to counter fluid loss. Adjust your intake to match these variables for sustained performance.

Investing in a reusable water bottle with measurement markers can help you monitor fluid intake during your workouts. For endurance athletes, hydration packs or bottles with straw systems provide easy access to fluids on the go.

Post-workout hydration is equally important for recovery. Weigh yourself before and after your workout to estimate fluid loss—each pound lost represents roughly 16 ounces of water that need replacing. Drinking water with added electrolytes can accelerate recovery and prevent delayed onset muscle soreness (DOMS).

By prioritizing hydration before, during, and after workouts, you safeguard your performance, support recovery, and optimize your training results. Incorporating these hydration strategies ensures you stay on track with both fitness and macro goals, paving the way for long-term success.

# Avoiding Hydration Pitfalls

## 3.1 The Dangers of Overhydration

Hydration is a cornerstone of health, yet drinking too much water can be just as harmful as not drinking enough. Overhydration, also known as water intoxication or hyponatremia, occurs when the body's sodium levels are diluted to dangerously low levels. Sodium, an essential electrolyte, regulates water balance, nerve function, and muscle contractions. When it becomes excessively diluted, the body can no longer function optimally, leading to symptoms such as headaches, nausea, confusion, and, in severe cases, life-threatening complications like seizures or coma.

This condition is most often seen in athletes who consume large amounts of water during prolonged activities without replenishing electrolytes. The excessive intake of water flushes out sodium, creating an imbalance that impairs cellular communication and organ function. However, overhydration is not limited to athletes. Misguided health practices that encourage drinking excessive amounts of water can lead to similar outcomes, particularly if electrolytes are not considered.

To avoid overhydration, it is important to understand your body's unique hydration needs. These are influenced by factors such as body weight, activity level, and environmental conditions. Rather than mindlessly drinking water, focus on listening to your body's signals. Thirst, for instance, is a natural indicator of hydration needs, though it should be supported by other measures such as monitoring urine color. Pale yellow urine suggests healthy hydration levels, whereas consistently clear urine may indicate you are drinking more than necessary.

Proper hydration practices also include balancing water intake with electrolyte replenishment. Including sodium and other electrolytes in your hydration routine ensures that your body retains the fluids it needs without diluting its mineral reserves. This balance is particularly crucial during intense physical activity or in hot weather when electrolyte loss through sweat is substantial. Staying mindful of this balance will help you stay safely hydrated without tipping into dangerous territory.

## 3.2 Dehydration and Hunger

Dehydration and hunger are often mistaken for one another because the body's signals for both can feel remarkably similar. When dehydrated, you might experience sensations like fatigue, irritability, and even a vague emptiness that is easy to misinterpret as a call for food. This confusion often leads people to snack unnecessarily when what their bodies really need is water.

The overlap between hunger and dehydration signals occurs because both are regulated by the hypothalamus, the part of the brain responsible for controlling thirst and appetite. When hydration levels drop, the hypothalamus may activate hunger cues instead of thirst, especially if you are already accustomed to irregular eating or drinking patterns. As a result, many people unknowingly eat extra calories, undermining their macro targets and fitness goals.

Staying consistently hydrated can mitigate this issue and clarify your body's signals. A useful approach is the "water first" method. When hunger arises unexpectedly, drinking a glass of water and waiting for about 15 to 20 minutes can help you determine if the sensation was true hunger or just thirst. More often than not, mild dehydration is the culprit behind perceived hunger.

Building hydration into your daily routine is also critical to preventing this confusion. Sipping water consistently throughout the day, rather than waiting for thirst to strike, ensures your body maintains an optimal balance. Additionally, consuming water-rich foods like fruits, vegetables, and soups provides both hydration and nourishment, reducing the likelihood of dehydration-driven hunger.

By understanding the close connection between hydration and hunger signals, you can make more informed decisions about when and what to eat. This awareness not only supports your hydration needs but also keeps your macro goals on track by minimizing unnecessary calorie intake.

## 3.3 Hydration and Macronutrient Absorption

The role of hydration extends far beyond simply quenching thirst; it is fundamental to how your body digests and absorbs macronutrients. Proteins, carbohydrates, and fats—the building blocks of your diet—require adequate water to be broken down, transported, and utilized effectively. Without sufficient hydration, these processes slow, reducing the efficiency of nutrient absorption and impairing your progress toward fitness goals.

Water is integral to digestion from the very beginning. In the stomach, water helps dissolve food and facilitates the action of digestive enzymes and stomach acids. For protein digestion, for instance, water ensures that amino acids—the components of muscle repair and growth—are properly extracted and absorbed. Similarly, carbohydrates, which provide the energy needed for both workouts and recovery, depend on water for their breakdown into glucose and subsequent delivery to cells.

Fats, often perceived as the most challenging macronutrient to digest, also rely on hydration. The production of bile, a digestive fluid critical for fat breakdown, is directly influenced by water availability. When hydration levels are low, bile production can decrease, slowing fat metabolism and potentially causing digestive discomfort.

Beyond digestion, water plays a vital role in transporting nutrients throughout the body. Once broken down, macronutrients are carried via the bloodstream to cells and tissues where they are needed. This process is water-dependent, meaning that even mild dehydration can impede nutrient delivery, leaving your muscles undernourished and less capable of recovery and growth.

To enhance macronutrient absorption, consider timing your hydration strategically around meals. Drinking water with your meals, rather than before or after, supports digestion without over-diluting stomach acids. Incorporating hydrating foods into your diet, such as cucumbers, oranges, or melons, can also provide additional fluids while contributing valuable vitamins and minerals.

In essence, hydration is inseparably linked to nutrient efficiency. By maintaining optimal water intake, you support not only the digestion and absorption of macronutrients but also their effective use in powering workouts, repairing muscles, and fueling your overall fitness journey.

# Grocery Lists and Meal Planning

## Building a Macro-Friendly Grocery List

### 1.1 Must-Have Macro-Friendly Foods

Building a macro-friendly grocery list is the foundation of any successful fitness or nutrition plan. The right foods ensure you hit your macronutrient targets while providing the essential nutrients needed for energy, recovery, and overall health. A well-thought-out list not only simplifies meal prep but also keeps you aligned with your fitness goals by reducing reliance on impulse buys or unbalanced meals.

Protein-rich foods should form the cornerstone of your list, as protein is essential for muscle repair and growth. Lean meats like chicken breast, turkey, and fish such as salmon or cod are excellent choices. For plant-based options, include tofu, tempeh, lentils, and beans. Eggs, Greek yogurt, and cottage cheese provide versatile, high-protein options suitable for any meal.

Carbohydrates are another crucial component. Prioritize complex carbs like brown rice, quinoa, oats, and sweet potatoes, which provide sustained energy and help replenish glycogen stores after workouts. For quick and convenient carb sources, consider whole-grain bread or wraps and a selection of fruits such as bananas, berries, and apples.

Healthy fats round out your macro-friendly shopping. Avocados, nuts, seeds, and olive oil deliver essential fatty acids that support brain function and hormone production. Fatty fish, such as mackerel or sardines, offers both protein and omega-3 fats, making it a dual-purpose addition to your list.

No macro-friendly grocery list is complete without a variety of vegetables. Non-starchy vegetables like spinach, kale, broccoli, and bell peppers provide essential vitamins, minerals, and fiber while being low in calories. These foods add bulk to meals, keeping you full and satisfied without affecting your macro balance.

By focusing on these staple items, you'll ensure that your pantry and fridge are stocked with nutrient-dense foods that support your fitness journey. With these essentials on hand, you'll have the tools to create balanced, macro-friendly meals with ease.

## 1.2 How to Read Nutrition Labels

Understanding how to read nutrition labels is an invaluable skill for anyone working toward macro-related goals. Labels provide the information needed to assess whether a product aligns with your protein, carbohydrate, and fat targets, making them a critical tool for making informed grocery decisions.

Start by examining the serving size at the top of the label. This indicates the portion for which all nutritional values are calculated. Often, products contain multiple servings per package, so it's important to adjust your calculations accordingly. For example, if a bag of granola lists 200 calories per serving but contains four servings, consuming the entire bag means you've consumed 800 calories.

Next, review the macronutrient breakdown. Proteins, carbohydrates, and fats are typically listed in grams per serving. Pay close attention to the sources of these macros. For carbohydrates, check the amount of fiber and sugar. High-fiber foods provide lasting energy and aid digestion, while high-sugar items may lead to energy crashes and excess calorie consumption.

Fats are categorized into saturated and unsaturated fats. Focus on products with higher unsaturated fat content, as these are heart-healthy and support overall well-being. Avoid foods high in trans fats, which are detrimental to cardiovascular health.

The ingredient list is another critical component. Ingredients are listed in descending order by weight, so the first few items often tell you the product's main components. Choose foods with minimal, recognizable ingredients to ensure they're less processed and nutrient-dense. For instance, a jar of peanut butter with just "peanuts and salt" is preferable to one with added sugars and oils.

Finally, consider the calorie count in the context of your daily macro goals. A food may appear healthy but can derail your plan if it's too calorie-dense for its macro content. For example, some protein bars contain high sugar levels, making them less ideal than whole-food options like grilled chicken or hard-boiled eggs.

By mastering nutrition labels, you'll have the confidence to make choices that align with your macro needs, ensuring your grocery trips are efficient and effective.

## 1.3 Shopping Smart on a Budget

Eating clean and hitting your macro goals doesn't have to break the bank. With strategic planning and smart shopping techniques, you can build a macro-friendly diet that's both nutritious and affordable. The key lies in choosing versatile ingredients, leveraging sales, and minimizing waste.

Begin by planning your meals for the week and creating a grocery list based on those meals. This not only reduces impulse purchases but also ensures you only buy what you need, preventing food waste. Sticking to your list will help you avoid unnecessary spending on items that don't align with your goals.

When it comes to proteins, budget-friendly options like chicken thighs, canned tuna, eggs, and legumes are excellent choices. Buying larger quantities, such as family packs of chicken or bulk ground turkey, can lower costs significantly. If freezer space permits, stock up during sales and portion out servings for future use. Plant-based protein sources, like lentils and beans, are not only affordable but also packed with fiber and other essential nutrients.

For carbohydrates, prioritize whole grains like oats, brown rice, and pasta, which are cost-effective and provide sustained energy. Potatoes are another inexpensive and versatile option, easily incorporated into a variety of dishes. Seasonal fruits and vegetables are typically cheaper than out-of-season produce and offer optimal freshness and taste. Frozen fruits and vegetables are also excellent choices, as they're often picked at peak ripeness and retain their nutrients.

Healthy fats can be pricey, but buying in bulk can help. Large containers of olive oil, bags of nuts, and tubs of seeds like chia or flaxseed offer long-term value. Spreading these out over multiple meals makes them more economical without sacrificing nutrition.

Shopping at discount grocers or farmers' markets can also yield significant savings. Additionally, consider generic brands, which often provide the same quality as name brands at a lower cost. Avoid pre-packaged or convenience foods, which tend to be more expensive and less macro-friendly.

By employing these strategies, you'll find that eating clean and hitting your macro goals is entirely achievable on a budget. Smart shopping habits not only save money but also empower you to make healthier, more consistent choices.

# Meal Planning for Success

## 2.1 Meal Prep Essentials

Meal prepping is a powerful tool for staying on track with your fitness and nutrition goals. By dedicating time to plan, prepare, and portion your meals for the week, you eliminate the guesswork of daily cooking, reduce reliance on unhealthy convenience foods, and ensure you hit your macronutrient targets consistently. With a few simple steps, meal prep can transform from an overwhelming task into a manageable and rewarding routine.

Begin with a clear plan. Take stock of your weekly schedule to identify the meals you'll need each day. For instance, if your evenings are busy, focus on preparing dinners in advance. Write out your meal plan and calculate the macronutrient breakdown for each meal, ensuring you stay within your goals for protein, carbs, and fats. This upfront planning is crucial to creating a balanced diet tailored to your needs.

Once your plan is set, build your grocery list based on the recipes and portions you'll prepare. Stick to versatile ingredients that can be used across multiple meals. For example, chicken breast can be grilled for salads, shredded for tacos, or paired with rice and vegetables for a complete meal. Having overlapping ingredients reduces waste and saves money.

When it's time to cook, set aside a dedicated block of time—typically one or two sessions per week—to prepare your meals. Invest in quality containers to portion out individual meals for easy grab-and-go convenience. Transparent, BPA-free containers make it easy to see what's inside, while portioned compartments help you control serving sizes.

Keep meals simple to start, focusing on recipes you're familiar with. As you get more comfortable, introduce variety to avoid meal fatigue. Incorporate fresh herbs, spices, and low-calorie sauces to enhance flavors without altering your macros.

Incorporating meal prep into your routine not only streamlines your week but also empowers you to make healthier choices consistently. With a little planning, you can eliminate stress, save time, and set yourself up for nutritional success.

## 2.2 Batch Cooking for Efficiency

Batch cooking is an excellent strategy for those seeking efficiency and consistency in their diet. By preparing large quantities of food in one session, you reduce the time spent cooking throughout the week while ensuring your meals align with your macronutrient goals. This approach is particularly beneficial for busy individuals balancing work, fitness, and other responsibilities.

The key to successful batch cooking is selecting recipes that are easy to scale and store well. Focus on staples like roasted chicken, grilled vegetables, rice, and stews, which maintain their flavor and texture over several days. Protein-rich dishes such as chili, baked salmon, or turkey meatballs are ideal for freezing and reheating without compromising quality.

Start by organizing your kitchen workspace. Ensure you have all the necessary tools, including cutting boards, knives, baking sheets, and large cooking pots or pans. Group similar tasks—such as chopping vegetables or marinating proteins—to streamline the process and maximize efficiency.

Cooking multiple items simultaneously is another time-saving technique. For instance, roast vegetables on one tray while baking chicken on another. Use a rice cooker or instant pot to prepare grains, freeing up your stovetop for other tasks. Having everything cooking at once reduces overall prep time and allows you to focus on portioning meals afterward.

Once the food is ready, portion it into individual containers based on your planned servings. Divide proteins, carbs, and fats evenly, ensuring each meal fits your macro targets. Label the containers with the meal name and date to maintain organization and avoid confusion later in the week.

Batch cooking also extends to snacks and side dishes. Preparing items like boiled eggs, overnight oats, or pre-cut fruit ensures you always have macro-friendly options on hand, reducing the temptation to reach for less nutritious alternatives.

By incorporating batch cooking into your routine, you save valuable time and energy while ensuring that your meals remain consistent and aligned with your goals. It's a practical approach that simplifies nutrition and enhances your ability to stay on track.

## 2.3 Flexibility in Meal Planning

While meal planning provides structure and consistency, it's important to leave room for flexibility. Life is unpredictable, and strict adherence to a rigid plan can sometimes lead to frustration or burnout. A flexible approach ensures you stay on track with your macros without feeling restricted, empowering you to adapt to changes and maintain a positive relationship with food.

Flexibility begins with understanding that plans are guidelines, not rules. If a planned meal doesn't appeal to you on a given day or if your schedule shifts unexpectedly, having alternative options ready ensures you don't deviate from your goals. Keep quick, macro-friendly staples like canned tuna, pre-cooked chicken, or protein shakes on hand for such situations.

Adjusting portion sizes is another aspect of flexibility. For instance, if you find yourself hungrier than usual after a workout, slightly increase your protein or carbohydrate portions to refuel effectively. Similarly, if you've eaten more than planned at one meal, balance it out by choosing lighter options later in the day. This dynamic approach allows you to respond to your body's needs without guilt or overcompensation.

Variety also plays a crucial role in maintaining flexibility. Rotate your meals weekly or biweekly to prevent monotony and ensure a broader intake of nutrients. Explore different cuisines and cooking methods to keep your diet exciting and satisfying. For example, swap grilled chicken and broccoli for a stir-fry or experiment with new seasonings and sauces.

Social events or dining out can also challenge a rigid meal plan. In such cases, focus on making mindful choices that align with your macros. Opt for lean proteins, vegetable-heavy dishes, and whole-grain sides where possible. If exact tracking isn't feasible, prioritize balance and portion control instead of striving for perfection.

By embracing flexibility in meal planning, you create a sustainable approach to nutrition that adapts to your lifestyle. This balance between structure and adaptability ensures long-term success without sacrificing enjoyment or convenience.

# Overcoming Grocery and Meal Prep Challenges

# 3.1 Time-Saving Tips

Time constraints are one of the most common obstacles to successful grocery shopping and meal preparation. However, with a few strategic adjustments, you can streamline the process and make meal prep more efficient without compromising on quality or nutrition.

The first step to saving time is creating a well-organized plan before heading to the grocery store. Write down a detailed list based on your weekly meal plan, grouping items by category—such as produce, proteins, and pantry staples—to minimize backtracking in the store. Many grocery stores now offer online shopping or curbside pickup, which can save hours each week while ensuring you stick to your list.

When it comes to meal prep, focus on multi-tasking. Cooking multiple components simultaneously is a game changer. For example, while roasting chicken and vegetables in the oven, boil grains like quinoa or rice on the stovetop. Use appliances such as slow cookers, pressure cookers, or air fryers to prepare hands-free dishes while you tackle other tasks.

Pre-cut and pre-washed ingredients can also significantly reduce prep time. Though they may cost slightly more, items like chopped vegetables or pre-cooked grains are worth the investment when time is tight. Batch cooking is another effective approach. Prepare large quantities of proteins, grains, and roasted vegetables, then mix and match them throughout the week for variety without extra effort.

Freezing meals and ingredients is another valuable time-saving technique. Cooking double portions of soups, stews, or casseroles allows you to freeze half for later weeks, ensuring you always have healthy, macro-friendly options on hand. Even individual ingredients like cooked chicken or sautéed vegetables can be portioned and frozen, ready to be incorporated into meals in minutes.

By implementing these strategies, you can reduce the time spent on shopping and meal prep while maintaining a consistent, healthy eating routine. Time-saving practices not only make meal prep manageable but also help build a sustainable system that supports your fitness goals.

## 3.2 Avoiding Meal Prep Fatigue

Meal prep can feel monotonous over time, especially when routines become too rigid or meals lack variety. This fatigue often leads to inconsistency, which can derail your progress. The key to staying motivated is keeping the process fresh, flexible, and aligned with your long-term goals.

A primary cause of meal prep fatigue is repetition. Eating the same meals day after day can make the process feel like a chore rather than a benefit. To combat this, introduce variety into your meal plans. Experiment with different cuisines, spices, and cooking techniques. For instance, swap plain grilled chicken for a flavorful curry or teriyaki stir-fry. Rotating recipes weekly or seasonally can keep your palate engaged and excited.

Setting realistic expectations is another way to stay consistent. While social media may glamorize elaborate meal prep setups, simplicity is often more sustainable. Focus on a few core dishes that you enjoy and are easy to prepare, rather than overwhelming yourself with complex recipes. Progress, not perfection, is what matters most.

Involving others can also make the process more enjoyable. If you live with family or friends, consider turning meal prep into a group activity. Splitting tasks like chopping vegetables or portioning meals can make the workload lighter and provide an opportunity for connection. Even solo meal preppers can find motivation by listening to music, podcasts, or audiobooks while cooking.

Another effective strategy is to remind yourself of the benefits. Meal prep saves time during the week, reduces stress, and ensures you stay on track with your macro goals. Keeping these benefits in mind can help reframe the process from a mundane task to an empowering routine that supports your fitness journey.

By approaching meal prep with creativity, flexibility, and mindfulness, you can overcome fatigue and maintain a consistent, enjoyable routine. This shift in perspective transforms meal prep from an obligation into a valuable tool for success.

## 3.3 Making Meal Prep Enjoyable

Meal prep doesn't have to feel like a chore; with the right mindset and strategies, it can become an enjoyable and even rewarding part of your weekly routine. By adding personal touches, focusing on creativity, and finding ways to make the process fun, you can turn meal prep into something you look forward to.

Start by creating a positive environment for meal prep. Choose a time when you feel relaxed and can dedicate your full attention to the task. Play your favorite music, put on an engaging podcast, or catch up on an audiobook while you cook. Creating an enjoyable atmosphere can make the process feel less like work and more like a moment of self-care.

Incorporate variety into your meals to keep things exciting. Explore new recipes or experiment with ingredients you've never tried before. For example, swap traditional pasta for zucchini noodles or quinoa for farro. Trying different cuisines, such as Mediterranean, Asian, or Latin-inspired dishes, can add a sense of adventure to your cooking. The more you enjoy what you eat, the more rewarding meal prep will feel.

Personalizing your meals is another way to add enjoyment. If you love spicy food, incorporate your favorite hot sauce or seasoning blend into dishes. If presentation excites you, invest in colorful containers or garnish your meals with fresh herbs and vibrant vegetables. Small touches can make a big difference in how much you appreciate the fruits of your labor.

Turning meal prep into a family or social activity is another way to boost enjoyment. Cooking with loved ones not only divides the workload but also creates an opportunity for bonding and shared creativity. If prepping solo, consider documenting your progress by taking photos of your meals or sharing tips with an online community, where you can find encouragement and inspiration.

All in all, celebrate your successes. When you see the benefits of your efforts—whether it's hitting macro goals, saving time, or simply enjoying delicious meals—it reinforces the value of meal prep. Over time, these positive associations can make meal prep an integral and enjoyable part of your lifestyle.

# Overcoming Common Nutrition Challenges

## Dealing with Cravings

### 1.1 Understanding Food Cravings

Food cravings are a universal experience, often tied to both physiological and psychological factors. Understanding the science behind cravings is the first step toward managing them effectively and maintaining a balanced relationship with food.

At their core, food cravings are influenced by the brain's reward system. When you consume foods high in sugar, fat, or salt, the brain releases dopamine, a chemical associated with pleasure and reward. Over time, frequent exposure to such foods can create a cycle of seeking them out to replicate this feeling. Emotional triggers also play a significant role, as stress, boredom, or fatigue can prompt cravings for comfort foods that provide a temporary sense of relief.

Hormonal imbalances may further contribute to cravings. For instance, low levels of serotonin, a neurotransmitter linked to mood regulation, can lead to a desire for carbohydrate-rich foods, which help boost serotonin production. Similarly, fluctuations in blood sugar levels can trigger cravings for sugary or high-carb snacks, especially if meals are inconsistent or unbalanced.

Nutrient deficiencies can also manifest as cravings. A craving for chocolate, for example, might indicate a magnesium deficiency, while a desire for salty foods could signal a lack of electrolytes. Identifying the root cause of your cravings can help address underlying issues and reduce their frequency.

Additionally, environmental and behavioral factors, such as exposure to advertisements or habitual snacking during certain activities, can create conditioned responses that reinforce cravings over time. Recognizing these triggers allows you to make conscious choices and regain control over your eating habits.

Understanding cravings is not about elimination but about awareness and balance. By identifying the physiological, psychological, and environmental factors at play, you can develop strategies to manage cravings without derailing your nutritional goals.

## 1.2 Strategies to Curb Cravings

Managing food cravings requires a combination of practical strategies and self-awareness. While cravings are natural, they don't have to control your eating habits. With the right approach, you can curb cravings effectively and maintain alignment with your nutrition plan.

The first step in managing cravings is maintaining balanced meals. Consuming a combination of protein, healthy fats, and fiber at each meal helps stabilize blood sugar levels, reducing the likelihood of sudden cravings. For instance, a breakfast of eggs, avocado, and whole-grain toast provides sustained energy and keeps hunger at bay.

Staying hydrated is equally important, as dehydration can sometimes mimic hunger or intensify cravings. Drinking water throughout the day ensures your body functions optimally and helps you differentiate between true hunger and a fleeting desire for food.

Planning ahead is another powerful tool. Stock your kitchen with macro-friendly snacks like nuts, Greek yogurt, or pre-cut vegetables to satisfy cravings without straying from your goals. Having healthier alternatives readily available makes it easier to resist less nutritious options.

Distraction techniques can also help. When a craving strikes, engage in an activity that shifts your focus, such as going for a walk, calling a friend, or practicing deep breathing. Cravings often fade after 15–20 minutes, especially when your mind is occupied.

Mindful eating practices are another effective strategy. Instead of acting on cravings immediately, take a moment to assess their origin. Ask yourself if you're truly hungry, stressed, or simply bored. If you decide to indulge, do so mindfully—savoring every bite—rather than eating mindlessly.

Lastly, ensure you're getting enough sleep. Sleep deprivation can disrupt hunger hormones like ghrelin and leptin, leading to increased cravings, particularly for sugary or high-calorie foods. Prioritizing quality sleep supports both your energy levels and your ability to manage cravings.

By implementing these strategies, you can navigate cravings with confidence, maintaining control over your diet while still enjoying food.

## 1.3 Balancing Indulgence and Macro Goals

Indulging in your favorite foods doesn't have to derail your nutrition goals. In fact, finding a balance between occasional indulgence and macro adherence is key to long-term sustainability. When approached mindfully, indulgence can enhance your relationship with food while supporting your overall progress.

The concept of moderation is central to this balance. Rather than labeling foods as "good" or "bad," recognize that all foods can fit into your diet when consumed in appropriate portions. For example, if you're craving chocolate, opt for a small square of dark chocolate instead of an entire bar. This approach satisfies the craving without significantly impacting your macros.

Incorporating indulgences into your plan proactively can also help. Allocate a small portion of your daily or weekly calories for treats you enjoy. For instance, you might include a scoop of ice cream as part of your post-dinner routine. By planning these moments, you reduce feelings of guilt and maintain control over your intake.

Flexible dieting, or the "80/20 rule," is another effective framework. This method involves consuming nutrient-dense, macro-aligned foods 80% of the time while allowing 20% for less structured choices. This balance supports both your physical and emotional well-being, making it easier to sustain your diet over time.

Mindful indulgence is about quality over quantity. Prioritize high-quality versions of your favorite treats, as they are often more satisfying. For example, a homemade pizza with fresh ingredients can be just as enjoyable as a greasy takeout option but with better control over macros.

It's also helpful to shift your mindset around indulgence. Instead of viewing it as a setback, consider it a normal and enjoyable part of life. When you approach treats with a positive attitude, you're less likely to spiral into guilt-driven overeating.

Ultimately, balancing indulgence and macro goals is about maintaining perspective. Occasional treats won't undo your progress as long as they are part of a broader pattern of mindful eating and consistent effort. By embracing moderation and flexibility, you create a sustainable approach to nutrition that supports both your goals and your happiness.

# Handling Social Situations

## 2.1 Dining Out Without Derailing Progress

Eating out doesn't have to mean sacrificing your nutrition goals. With the right strategies, you can enjoy dining out while staying on track with your macros, proving that flexibility and discipline can coexist.

Start by reviewing the menu ahead of time. Most restaurants have their menus online, allowing you to plan your meal in advance. Look for dishes rich in lean protein, such as grilled chicken, fish, or steak, paired with vegetables or whole grains. Avoid anything labeled "crispy," "fried," or "smothered," as these are often calorie-dense and low in nutritional value.

When ordering, don't hesitate to customize your meal. Ask for sauces and dressings on the side, request steamed vegetables instead of fries, or swap out carb-heavy sides for a salad. Most restaurants are happy to accommodate such requests, and taking control of your order allows you to better manage your macros.

Portion control is also key. Restaurant servings are often oversized, making it easy to overeat. Consider splitting your meal with a dining companion or asking for a to-go box at the start of the meal and saving half for later. This not only helps you stay within your calorie goals but also provides an extra meal for the next day.

Drinks are another area where hidden calories lurk. Stick to water, unsweetened tea, or sparkling water with lemon instead of sugary sodas or calorie-laden cocktails. If you choose to indulge in alcohol, opt for lower-calorie options like a glass of wine or a vodka soda, and drink in moderation.

Finally, embrace the mindset that dining out is about the experience, not just the food. Focus on the company, the ambiance, and the conversation. By shifting your attention away from indulgent eating and toward the overall experience, you can enjoy the outing without veering off track.

Dining out is not an all-or-nothing situation. With mindful choices and a proactive approach, you can navigate restaurant meals with confidence, allowing you to enjoy social occasions while staying committed to your fitness journey.

## 2.2 Navigating Holidays and Parties

Festive events like holidays and parties are a common stumbling block for those following a macro-based diet. However, with advanced planning and mindful strategies, you can celebrate without compromising your progress.

Preparation is your strongest ally. Before the event, eat a balanced meal containing protein, fiber, and healthy fats to stabilize your blood sugar and curb excessive hunger. This reduces the temptation to overindulge in calorie-dense party foods. Hydration also plays a role; drinking water before and during the event helps you feel fuller and keeps dehydration-induced cravings at bay.

When faced with a buffet or spread, start with a survey. Take a moment to assess the options before filling your plate. Prioritize protein-rich foods like turkey, shrimp, or grilled chicken and pair them with vegetables or lighter sides. Limit portions of carb-heavy or fried items, and skip foods you don't genuinely enjoy. This mindful approach allows you to indulge selectively while maintaining control.

Portion awareness is essential. Opt for smaller servings to sample different dishes without overeating. Use a smaller plate if possible, as this visually limits how much you can pile on. If you're tempted to go back for seconds, take a break and assess your hunger first—often, the urge to refill diminishes after a few minutes.

Alcohol is another challenge during festive events. Stick to clear spirits with zero-calorie mixers, wine, or light beer to minimize calorie intake. Alternate alcoholic drinks with water to stay hydrated and slow down your consumption.

If you're hosting or contributing to the meal, use this opportunity to prepare a dish that aligns with your macros. Healthy options like roasted vegetables, protein-packed dips, or a low-calorie dessert ensure you have at least one macro-friendly option on the table.

Finally, be kind to yourself. Holidays and parties are about connection and joy, not perfection. If you go slightly over your macros, remember that one day won't undo your progress. Get back on track with your next meal and view the event as a moment to enjoy rather than a setback.

## 2.3 Staying on Track While Traveling

Traveling presents unique challenges for maintaining macro discipline, but it also offers opportunities for growth and adaptability. By planning ahead and staying mindful, you can manage your nutrition goals without feeling restricted during your journey.

Preparation begins before you leave. Pack macro-friendly snacks like protein bars, nuts, dried fruit, or jerky to avoid relying on less nutritious convenience foods. If you're flying, these portable options are easy to carry and help you resist high-calorie airport meals. For road trips, consider packing a cooler with pre-made meals or snacks to keep you fueled on the go.

Research is another crucial step. Familiarize yourself with dining options at your destination, especially if you're staying in a new city or country. Apps like MyFitnessPal and Yelp can help you find restaurants with healthier options and provide nutritional information. If possible, book accommodations with a kitchenette so you can prepare some of your meals and maintain control over your diet.

When dining out while traveling, apply the same principles you use at home: prioritize lean proteins, vegetables, and whole grains, and avoid fried or overly processed items. If you're unsure about portion sizes or ingredients, don't hesitate to ask the staff for details or modifications.

Hydration is especially important during travel, as long flights, increased activity, and unfamiliar climates can lead to dehydration. Carry a refillable water bottle to ensure you're drinking enough throughout the day.

Finally, embrace flexibility. Travel often involves unexpected changes, from delayed flights to spontaneous meals. Instead of striving for perfection, aim for balance. If one meal is indulgent, make the next one lighter and more aligned with your macros. Incorporate physical activity—whether it's walking through a new city or using the hotel gym—to offset any dietary indulgences.

Travel is an opportunity to explore new environments and cultures, and food is often a big part of that experience. By adopting a balanced approach, you can enjoy your journey while staying committed to your long-term goals.

## Managing Mental Blocks

## 3.1 Staying Consistent in the Face of Stress

Stress is an inevitable part of life, but its impact on your nutrition goals doesn't have to be. The challenge lies not in avoiding stress, but in managing how it affects your behaviors, especially when it comes to maintaining consistency with your nutrition.

When you're stressed, your body enters a fight-or-flight response, often leading to emotional eating or poor food choices as a way to cope. This might involve reaching for sugary snacks or comfort foods that provide a temporary sense of relief but can quickly derail your progress. To counter this, it's essential to develop stress management techniques that support your well-being while keeping you on track with your goals.

One effective approach is mindfulness. Taking a few moments to breathe deeply and reconnect with your body can reduce the intensity of stress and prevent impulsive food choices. Practicing mindfulness can also help you distinguish between emotional hunger and physical hunger, allowing you to make more intentional food decisions.

In addition to mindfulness, planning ahead can be a game-changer. When life gets chaotic, having a prepped meal or a quick, healthy snack on hand ensures you won't default to unhealthy options out of convenience. Consistent meal prepping and maintaining a routine can provide stability amidst stress, giving you a sense of control over your eating habits.

Exercise is another powerful tool. Physical activity helps reduce stress hormones like cortisol while boosting mood-enhancing endorphins. Whether it's a short walk or a more intense workout, regular movement not only supports your fitness goals but also improves your mental resilience, making it easier to stay focused on your nutrition.

By addressing stress proactively, you build a foundation that allows you to stay consistent with your nutrition, no matter what challenges arise. It's not about eliminating stress, but about learning to navigate it without letting it derail your journey.

## 3.2 Overcoming Guilt and Perfectionism

In a world where perfectionism is often glorified, it's easy to fall into the trap of guilt when things don't go exactly as planned. Whether you indulge in an off-plan meal or miss a workout, these moments don't have to spiral into feelings of failure. Instead, they can serve as valuable learning opportunities.

The first step in overcoming guilt is understanding that no one is perfect. Even the most disciplined individuals experience slip-ups. Perfectionism sets an unrealistic standard that ultimately causes more harm than good. Rather than focusing on what went wrong, shift your attention to what you can do next.

It's helpful to reframe your mindset around mistakes. Rather than seeing a deviation from your plan as a setback, consider it a part of the process. Life is unpredictable, and being able to adapt without guilt or shame is essential for long-term success. If you overeat at a social event, for example, don't let it define the rest of your day or week. Acknowledge the moment, learn from it, and move on.

Another key aspect of overcoming guilt is practicing self-compassion. Instead of harshly judging yourself, treat yourself with the same kindness you would offer a friend in the same situation. Acknowledging that it's okay to be imperfect allows you to maintain balance and stay on track without internalizing negative feelings.

Building resilience against perfectionism also involves creating a flexible approach to your nutrition goals. Rather than adhering to rigid rules, allow space for occasional indulgences. Focus on the bigger picture, and remember that long-term success is built on consistency, not perfection.

In the journey of nutrition and fitness, setbacks are inevitable. The way you respond to them defines your path forward. By letting go of guilt and embracing flexibility, you create the mental space to continue moving forward with confidence.

## 3.3 Developing a Positive Relationship with Food

A positive relationship with food is foundational to long-term health and fitness success. Far too often, food is viewed through a lens of restriction, guilt, or fear. But food, in its many forms, is fuel—nourishing our bodies and supporting our overall well-being. Developing a healthy mental outlook on eating is crucial for maintaining a sustainable approach to your goals.

The first step toward a positive relationship with food is to stop viewing it as the enemy. Many people see "healthy eating" as synonymous with deprivation or restriction. In reality, eating nutritiously should be about nourishing your body and feeling good, not about punishing yourself or following a strict set of rules.

Shift your focus from dieting to adopting a balanced, inclusive approach. Instead of labeling foods as "good" or "bad," recognize that all foods have a place in your diet. Healthy eating doesn't require perfection—it requires variety, enjoyment, and balance. By allowing yourself the flexibility to indulge in your favorite foods occasionally, you can remove the stigma and guilt that often accompany eating.

Another key aspect is learning to listen to your body. Intuitive eating, which involves tuning into your hunger and fullness cues, helps you reconnect with your natural appetite rhythms. When you eat mindfully and with intention, you begin to distinguish between true hunger and emotional cravings. This practice reduces the likelihood of overeating and fosters a healthier, more respectful relationship with food.

In addition, adopting a mindset of gratitude toward food can shift your perspective. Instead of focusing on calories or macros, appreciate the nourishment that food provides and the role it plays in your health and vitality. This attitude helps cultivate a sense of respect for the food you consume and the impact it has on your well-being.

Lastly, it's important to let go of the all-or-nothing mentality. Life is full of spontaneous moments—celebrations, holidays, social gatherings—and these moments should be embraced, not feared. A positive relationship with food means finding harmony between your health goals and your life's pleasures.

By developing a healthy, balanced relationship with food, you empower yourself to make choices that align with your body's needs without guilt or stress. The key is to approach eating as an opportunity for nourishment, enjoyment, and self-care—leading to a more sustainable and fulfilling path to health and fitness.

# Advanced Techniques for Fine-Tuning Macros

## Using Advanced Tracking Tools

### 1.1 Macronutrient Calculators: Introducing Tools to Refine Tracking

In the pursuit of optimal health and physique, precision in dietary intake is paramount. Macronutrient calculators have emerged as indispensable tools, enabling individuals to tailor their nutrition according to specific goals—be it weight loss, muscle gain, or maintenance. These calculators consider variables such as age, weight, height, activity level, and objectives to provide personalized macronutrient distributions.

One notable example is the macro calculator offered by Legion Athletics, which assists users in determining their ideal caloric and macronutrient needs based on personal data. Similarly, the calculator provided by Bodybuilding.com utilizes the Mifflin-St Jeor equation, a widely recognized method for estimating basal metabolic rate, to offer tailored macronutrient recommendations.

The accuracy of these calculators is enhanced when users input precise and current data. Regular updates to personal information, such as changes in weight or activity level, are crucial for maintaining the relevance of the recommendations. Additionally, understanding the rationale behind the suggested macronutrient ratios can empower individuals to make informed dietary choices that align with their physiological needs and performance goals.

While macronutrient calculators provide a solid foundation, they should be used as part of a comprehensive nutritional strategy. Factors such as micronutrient intake, meal timing, and individual metabolic responses also play significant roles in overall health and performance. Therefore, combining the use of these calculators with professional guidance from nutritionists or dietitians can lead to more effective and sustainable outcomes.

All this implies that, macronutrient calculators serve as valuable tools for individuals seeking to fine-tune their dietary intake with precision. By providing personalized macronutrient distributions, they facilitate informed decision-making and support the achievement of specific health and fitness objectives. However, their effectiveness is maximized when integrated into a holistic nutritional approach that considers the full spectrum of dietary and lifestyle factors.

## 1.2 Progress Monitoring Beyond the Scale: Tracking Body Composition

Achieving health and fitness goals extends beyond mere weight measurement; understanding body composition offers a more comprehensive insight into physical health. Body composition analysis differentiates between fat mass, lean muscle mass, bone density, and water content, providing a nuanced perspective that the scale alone cannot offer.

Traditional methods like Body Mass Index (BMI) offer a general assessment but often fail to distinguish between muscle and fat, potentially misclassifying individuals with higher muscle mass as overweight. Advanced techniques such as Dual-Energy X-ray Absorptiometry (DEXA) scans, bioelectrical impedance analysis, and skinfold measurements provide more accurate assessments of body composition. These methods enable individuals to track changes in muscle mass and fat distribution, offering a clearer picture of health and fitness progress.

Regular monitoring of body composition is particularly beneficial for those engaged in strength training or muscle-building programs. An increase in muscle mass accompanied by fat loss may not result in significant weight change, but it indicates positive changes in body composition. Understanding these shifts can enhance motivation and inform necessary adjustments to training and nutrition plans.

Incorporating body composition analysis into regular health assessments allows for a more personalized approach to fitness and nutrition. It enables the identification of specific areas for improvement, such as increasing muscle mass or reducing visceral fat, and facilitates the development of targeted strategies to address these areas.

Most importantly, monitoring body composition provides a deeper understanding of physical health beyond what the scale can reveal. By focusing on the quality of weight—distinguishing between muscle and fat—individuals can make more informed decisions about their health and fitness journeys, leading to more effective and personalized outcomes.

## 1.3 Leveraging Fitness Trackers: Utilizing Wearable for Enhanced Insights

In the digital age, fitness trackers have become essential companions for individuals striving to optimize their health and performance. These wearable devices offer real-time data on various metrics, including heart rate, activity levels, sleep patterns, and even macronutrient tracking, providing users with actionable insights to fine-tune their fitness regimens.

Modern fitness trackers, such as the Apple Watch Series 10 and the Garmin Venu Sq 2, integrate advanced sensors capable of monitoring physiological parameters with remarkable accuracy. These devices can track energy expenditure, monitor heart rate variability, and assess sleep quality, offering a comprehensive overview of an individual's health status.

The data collected by fitness trackers can be synchronized with nutrition apps like MyFitnessPal, enabling seamless logging of dietary intake and macronutrient distribution. This integration allows users to correlate their nutritional habits with physical activity levels, facilitating more informed decisions regarding diet and exercise. For instance, understanding the relationship between caloric intake and expenditure can aid in achieving specific body composition goals.

Beyond activity tracking, many wearables offer features that monitor stress levels, provide guided breathing exercises, and deliver personalized feedback based on individual health data. These functionalities support holistic well-being by addressing both physical and mental health aspects.

However, the effectiveness of fitness trackers depends on user engagement and accurate data interpretation. Regularly reviewing the collected data and adjusting lifestyle choices accordingly is crucial for achieving desired outcomes. Additionally, while fitness trackers provide valuable insights, they should complement, not replace, professional medical advice and personalized training programs.

Look, leveraging fitness trackers enhances the ability to monitor and adjust health and fitness parameters in real-time. By providing detailed insights into various physiological metrics, these wearables empower individuals to make informed decisions, optimize their training routines, and achieve their health objectives more efficiently.

# Fine-Tuning for Peak Performance

## 2.1 Manipulating Carbs for Performance: Exploring Carb Cycling and Advanced Techniques

Achieving peak athletic performance often requires strategic dietary adjustments, particularly concerning carbohydrate intake. Carb cycling, a method involving planned variations in carbohydrate consumption, has gained prominence among athletes and fitness enthusiasts aiming to optimize energy levels and enhance performance. This approach entails alternating between high-carb and low-carb days, typically synchronized with training intensity. On days of intense training, increased carbohydrate intake replenishes glycogen stores, providing the necessary fuel for strenuous workouts. Conversely, on rest or low-intensity days, reducing carbohydrate consumption can promote fat utilization for energy, potentially aiding in body composition goals.

Implementing carb cycling requires careful planning and individualization. Athletes might adopt various patterns, such as several consecutive low-carb days followed by high-carb days, depending on their specific goals and training schedules. This strategic manipulation of carbohydrate intake can enhance metabolic flexibility, allowing the body to efficiently switch between fuel sources based on availability and demand.

However, it's essential to approach carb cycling with caution. Individual responses can vary, and factors such as the type of sport, training intensity, and personal health status should guide carbohydrate manipulation. Consulting with a registered dietitian or nutrition expert can provide personalized guidance, ensuring that carb cycling aligns with specific performance objectives and health considerations.

Above all, carb cycling offers a structured method to tailor carbohydrate intake in alignment with training demands, potentially enhancing energy utilization and performance outcomes. When implemented thoughtfully, it serves as a valuable tool in an athlete's nutritional strategy, contributing to the achievement of peak performance.

## 2.2 Protein Timing and Distribution: Optimizing Intake for Muscle Growth

Protein plays a pivotal role in muscle repair and growth, making its timing and distribution crucial for athletes seeking hypertrophy. Recent research suggests that consuming protein in proximity to training sessions can enhance muscle protein synthesis. The concept of an "anabolic window," traditionally believed to be a narrow timeframe post-exercise, has evolved. Current evidence indicates that this window may extend several hours post-training, allowing for more flexibility in nutrient timing.

Distributing protein intake evenly across meals throughout the day is also beneficial. Aim to include 20-30 grams of high-quality protein per meal to maintain a positive protein balance, supporting continuous muscle repair and growth. This approach ensures a steady supply of amino acids, the building blocks of muscle tissue, facilitating optimal recovery and adaptation from training stimuli.

Incorporating protein-rich snacks between meals and considering a presleep protein source can further support muscle protein synthesis during overnight recovery. Casein protein, found in dairy products like cottage cheese, is a slow-digesting protein that provides a sustained release of amino acids, making it an excellent choice before bedtime.

It's important to note that individual protein needs may vary based on factors such as body weight, training intensity, and overall dietary intake. Consulting with a sports nutritionist can provide personalized recommendations to optimize protein intake, timing, and distribution, aligning with specific muscle growth and performance goals.

It's very key to note that, strategic protein timing and distribution are integral components of a nutrition plan aimed at maximizing muscle growth. By ensuring adequate protein intake around training sessions and evenly throughout the day, athletes can enhance muscle protein synthesis, leading to improved strength and hypertrophy outcomes.

## 2.3 Adjusting Fats for Energy and Hormonal Balance: Tailoring Intake to Specific Needs

Dietary fats are essential macronutrients that play a significant role in energy provision and hormone production. For athletes, understanding how to adjust fat intake to meet specific energy demands and support hormonal health is crucial.

Fats serve as a dense energy source, particularly beneficial during prolonged, low to moderate-intensity activities where the body relies more heavily on fat oxidation. Incorporating healthy fats, such as those from avocados, nuts, seeds, and olive oil, can provide sustained energy, supporting endurance performance.

Beyond energy, fats are integral to hormone synthesis, including testosterone and estrogen, which are vital for muscle development and overall health. Maintaining adequate fat intake ensures the body has the necessary substrates for hormone production, influencing muscle growth, recovery, and immune function.

The general recommendation for athletes is to derive approximately 20-35% of total daily caloric intake from fats, focusing on unsaturated fats while limiting saturated and trans fats. However, individual requirements may vary based on factors such as training intensity, body composition goals, and metabolic health. For instance, athletes undergoing intense training phases may benefit from slightly higher fat intake to meet increased energy demands without excessively elevating carbohydrate or protein consumption.

It's also important to consider the timing of fat intake. Consuming high-fat meals immediately before high-intensity workouts may not be ideal, as fats digest slowly and could cause gastrointestinal discomfort. Instead, scheduling fat-rich meals at times distant from training sessions can help avoid potential digestive issues while still reaping the benefits of dietary fats.

After all, adjusting dietary fat intake in accordance with individual energy needs and hormonal health is a nuanced yet vital aspect of an athlete's nutrition strategy. By selecting appropriate fat sources, adhering to recommended intake ranges, and timing consumption effectively, athletes can support both their performance and overall well-being.

# Overcoming Plateaus and Breaking Through Limits

# 3.1 Recognizing Plateaus in Progress: Identifying When You're Stuck

In any fitness journey, encountering a plateau—a period where progress stalls despite consistent effort—is a common and often frustrating experience. Recognizing the signs of a plateau is the first step toward overcoming it. Common indicators include a halt in weight loss or muscle gain, diminished strength improvements, or a lack of progression in endurance levels. These stagnations occur even when adhering to established workout routines and dietary plans.

Several factors can contribute to plateaus. The body is remarkably adaptive; over time, it becomes efficient at performing repetitive exercises, leading to fewer calories burned and reduced muscle engagement. Additionally, metabolic adaptations can occur, where the body's energy expenditure decreases as weight is lost, making further progress challenging. External factors such as inadequate sleep, elevated stress levels, or insufficient recovery time can also impede progress.

To accurately identify a plateau, it's essential to maintain detailed records of workouts, dietary intake, and physical changes. Tracking tools and apps can assist in monitoring these variables, providing tangible data to assess progress. Regular self-assessment, including measuring body composition and performance metrics, offers insights into whether you're truly at a standstill or experiencing a natural fluctuation. Seeking feedback from fitness professionals can also provide an objective perspective, helping to identify areas that may require adjustment.

Recognizing a plateau is not a sign of failure but rather an opportunity to re-evaluate and adjust your approach. Understanding that plateaus are a natural part of the fitness journey can foster a proactive mindset, encouraging the implementation of new strategies to reignite progress.

## 3.2 Adjusting Macros to Push Through: Strategies to Break Through Stagnation

Once a plateau is identified, adjusting macronutrient (macro) intake can be an effective strategy to overcome stagnation. The body's nutritional needs evolve with changes in weight, muscle mass, and activity levels; therefore, recalibrating your diet to align with current goals is crucial.

One approach involves modifying caloric intake. As weight decreases, the body's energy requirements diminish, necessitating a reduction in calorie consumption to continue weight loss. Conversely, if muscle gain is the goal, a slight increase in calories, emphasizing protein intake, can provide the necessary resources for muscle synthesis. It's important to adjust calories gradually to prevent metabolic disruptions.

Altering the ratios of macronutrients—proteins, carbohydrates, and fats—can also stimulate progress. For instance, increasing protein intake supports muscle repair and growth, while adjusting carbohydrate levels can influence energy availability and fat metabolism. In some cases, incorporating techniques like carb cycling, which involves alternating high and low carbohydrate days, can enhance metabolic flexibility and break through plateaus.

Implementing these dietary adjustments should be done thoughtfully. Consulting with a registered dietitian or nutrition expert can provide personalized guidance, ensuring that changes in macro distribution are tailored to your specific needs and goals. Regular monitoring of your body's response to these adjustments is essential, allowing for further refinements based on progress and feedback.

Strategic modifications to macronutrient intake can serve as a catalyst for overcoming plateaus. By aligning your diet with your current physiological state and fitness objectives, you can reignite progress and continue advancing toward your goals.

## 3.3 The Importance of Patience and Consistency: Persevering Through Slow Progress

In the pursuit of fitness goals, patience and consistency are indispensable virtues. Progress is often incremental, and the journey is rarely linear. Embracing this reality fosters a sustainable and resilient approach to health and fitness.

Consistency in adhering to workout routines and nutritional plans establishes the foundation for success. Regular exercise and mindful eating habits lead to cumulative benefits over time, even when immediate results are not apparent. It's important to recognize that the body requires time to adapt to new stimuli, whether it's a change in exercise intensity or dietary adjustments. Maintaining consistency during these adaptation periods is crucial for long-term progress.

Patience plays a critical role in managing expectations and sustaining motivation. Understanding that setbacks and plateaus are natural components of the fitness journey can prevent discouragement. Cultivating patience allows for a focus on long-term objectives rather than immediate gratification, promoting a healthier relationship with fitness and self-improvement.

To bolster patience and consistency, setting realistic and attainable goals is essential. Breaking down larger objectives into smaller, manageable milestones provides a sense of achievement and keeps motivation levels high. Additionally, seeking support from fitness communities or professionals can offer encouragement and accountability, reinforcing commitment during challenging times.

Let's be frank, patience and consistency are the cornerstones of overcoming plateaus and achieving sustained fitness success. By steadfastly adhering to your fitness regimen and maintaining a patient outlook, you can navigate the inevitable challenges of the journey and emerge stronger and more accomplished.

# Building Lasting Habits for Success

## Creating Sustainable Routines

### 1.1 Designing Habits That Stick: Crafting Enduring Routines

Embarking on a fitness journey requires more than just initial enthusiasm; it demands the creation of sustainable habits that endure over time. The foundation of such habits lies in understanding your core motivations. Begin by clearly defining your goals and the underlying reasons driving them. This self-awareness not only provides direction but also fuels the persistence needed to maintain new routines.

Once your objectives are clear, it's essential to start with manageable changes. Attempting to overhaul your lifestyle overnight can lead to overwhelm and burnout. Instead, focus on small, incremental adjustments that seamlessly integrate into your daily life. This approach not only makes the process less daunting but also increases the likelihood of long-term adherence.

Creating an environment conducive to your new habits is equally important. Design your surroundings to minimize obstacles and reinforce positive behaviors. For instance, preparing your gym attire the night before can eliminate morning decision fatigue, making it easier to commit to your workout routine. Similarly, keeping nutritious snacks accessible can encourage healthier eating choices throughout the day.

Consistency is the cornerstone of habit formation. Engaging in your chosen activity at the same time each day can reinforce the behavior, gradually embedding it into your routine. Over time, these actions become second nature, reducing the reliance on willpower and making the habit more sustainable.

It's also beneficial to anticipate potential challenges and plan accordingly. By identifying possible obstacles in advance, you can develop strategies to overcome them, ensuring that temporary setbacks don't derail your progress. This proactive approach fosters resilience and adaptability, key components in maintaining lasting habits.

At this instance, designing habits that stick involves a thoughtful and deliberate approach. By understanding your motivations, starting small, optimizing your environment, maintaining consistency, and planning for challenges, you lay the groundwork for routines that not only support your fitness goals but also become an integral part of your lifestyle.

## 1.2 Making Macro Tracking Automatic: Integrating Seamless Nutritional Monitoring

Incorporating macronutrient (macro) tracking into your daily routine can significantly enhance your fitness outcomes. To make this practice second nature, begin by selecting a tracking method that aligns with your lifestyle. Whether it's a mobile app, a spreadsheet, or a handwritten journal, the key is to choose a tool that you find intuitive and convenient.

Once you've chosen your tracking method, establish a consistent routine for logging your meals. Setting aside a specific time each day—such as after each meal or during a quiet evening moment—can help reinforce the habit. By making tracking a regular part of your schedule, it becomes an automatic aspect of your daily life.

To further streamline the process, consider pre-planning your meals. By deciding in advance what you'll eat, you can enter the information into your tracking tool ahead of time, reducing the likelihood of deviations and ensuring nutritional compliance. This proactive approach not only simplifies tracking but also aids in making healthier food choices.

It's also important to be flexible and forgiving with yourself. Perfection isn't the goal; consistency is. If you miss a day or indulge in an unplanned treat, don't be discouraged. Acknowledge it and refocus on your tracking the next day. This mindset fosters a healthy relationship with food and tracking, preventing feelings of guilt or frustration.

By applying these strategies, macro tracking can become an effortless and automatic part of your daily routine, supporting your fitness goals without becoming a source of stress or inconvenience.

## 1.3 Reassessing Goals and Habits Regularly: Staying Aligned with Your Objectives

The journey toward fitness and health is dynamic, necessitating regular reflection and adjustment. Periodically reassessing your goals and habits ensures they remain aligned with your evolving aspirations and circumstances.

Begin by scheduling regular evaluations of your progress. This could be monthly or quarterly, depending on your preferences. During these assessments, reflect on your achievements, challenges, and any changes in your personal or professional life that may impact your fitness journey.

Consider whether your current habits are effectively contributing to your goals. If you find certain routines are no longer serving you, don't hesitate to modify or replace them. Flexibility is crucial in maintaining a sustainable and enjoyable fitness regimen.

Additionally, as you progress, your goals may evolve. What was once a primary objective may become less relevant as you achieve milestones and set new aspirations. Regularly updating your goals keeps you motivated and focused, providing a clear direction for your efforts.

Engaging with a fitness community or seeking feedback from a coach can offer valuable insights during these reassessments. External perspectives can highlight areas for improvement that you might overlook and provide encouragement to continue striving toward your objectives.

Making a habit of reassessing your goals and routines ensures that your fitness journey remains purposeful and aligned with your current needs and desires. This practice fosters continuous growth and adaptation, key elements in achieving long-term success.

# Staying Accountable

## 2.1 Tracking and Journaling for Accountability: The Role of Self-Reflection

One of the most effective ways to maintain accountability in your fitness journey is through consistent tracking and journaling. Writing down your goals, progress, and challenges creates a tangible record of your efforts, helping you stay aligned with your objectives. Journaling fosters self-awareness by encouraging you to reflect on your habits, understand your triggers, and identify areas for improvement.

Start by setting aside a few minutes each day to document your activities. This can include logging your workouts, meals, mood, and energy levels. Many find that pairing this habit with existing routines—like reflecting before bed or during a morning coffee break—makes it easier to sustain. Using physical journals, digital apps, or spreadsheets depends on your preference, but the key is consistency.

Moreover, journaling helps you track patterns over time. If you notice recurring obstacles, such as skipping workouts after stressful workdays, you can address them proactively by planning alternative strategies, like scheduling exercise earlier in the day. Similarly, recognizing positive trends—like increased energy after balanced meals—reinforces good habits.

In addition to tracking physical progress, journaling also supports mental well-being. Writing about your challenges and successes can reduce stress and foster a positive outlook. This process transforms journaling into more than a tool for accountability; it becomes a source of motivation and self-discovery.

## 2.2 Finding an Accountability Partner: Strengthening Commitment Through Support

While self-accountability is essential, sharing your goals with an accountability partner can significantly enhance your commitment. This person could be a friend, family member, or fitness coach who encourages your progress and helps you stay on track.

Accountability partners provide external motivation and perspective. They can check in on your progress, celebrate your wins, and offer constructive feedback when you face challenges. Knowing that someone else is invested in your success adds an extra layer of responsibility, making it less likely for you to skip workouts or veer off your meal plan.

Choosing the right partner is crucial. Look for someone who shares similar values and goals or has a genuine interest in your well-being. Communication is key—agree on how often you'll check in and the type of support you both need. For some, this might mean daily texts or weekly progress reviews, while others may prefer occasional catch-ups.

Online communities and fitness groups can also serve as accountability networks, especially if you don't have someone nearby. Platforms like social media or fitness forums connect you with like-minded individuals who can cheer you on and share insights.

The partnership doesn't just benefit you; it's mutually motivating. Your accountability partner may also strive toward their own goals, creating a collaborative dynamic where both parties grow and succeed together.

## 2.3 Celebrating Milestones: Acknowledging Progress for Sustained Motivation

Recognizing your achievements, no matter how small, is an essential aspect of staying accountable. Celebrating milestones reinforces the effort you've put in and reminds you that progress is being made, even if the ultimate goal is still ahead.

Milestones can take many forms, such as reaching a specific weight, completing a workout program, or sticking to your macro plan for a month. By setting both short-term and long-term goals, you create opportunities for frequent celebrations, which help maintain momentum and motivation.

When celebrating, choose rewards that align with your fitness journey. For example, treat yourself to new workout gear, a healthy meal at your favorite restaurant, or a relaxing spa day. These rewards reinforce your dedication and keep you excited about the process.

It's also valuable to share your successes with others. Posting about your achievements in a fitness group or discussing them with your accountability partner can boost your confidence and inspire others.

However, it's essential to avoid perfectionism during this process. Progress is rarely linear, and setbacks are part of any journey. Celebrating milestones reminds you that every step forward is significant, even if it's not flawless.

By tracking progress, leaning on support, and celebrating wins, you'll not only stay accountable but also enjoy the journey, ensuring lasting success in your fitness and health endeavors.

# Overcoming Setbacks and Staying Motivated

## 3.1 Handling Failures Without Giving Up: Building Resilience Through Challenges

Setbacks are inevitable in any fitness journey, but they don't have to derail your progress. Learning to handle failures with resilience is a skill that transforms temporary missteps into opportunities for growth. Whether it's missing a workout, indulging in unhealthy meals, or experiencing a plateau, the key is to view setbacks as part of the process rather than a sign of failure.

Start by reframing how you perceive setbacks. Instead of seeing them as a step backward, consider them as valuable feedback. For example, if you find yourself consistently skipping workouts, examine the reasons behind it. Is your schedule too packed, or are you choosing exercises that you don't enjoy? Identifying the root cause helps you develop solutions that prevent similar challenges in the future.

Additionally, practice self-compassion. Berating yourself for a missed goal only adds stress and can make it harder to regain momentum. Remind yourself that progress isn't linear and that everyone encounters obstacles along the way. Focus on what you can do next rather than dwelling on what went wrong.

Having a plan for when setbacks occur is also essential. Create a list of actionable steps to get back on track, such as revisiting your goals, adjusting your routines, or seeking support from a coach or accountability partner. By viewing setbacks as temporary and manageable, you cultivate a mindset that prioritizes perseverance over perfection.

## 3.2 Reinforcing Motivation Through Small Wins: Harnessing Momentum for Long-Term Success

Motivation often wanes during long-term fitness pursuits, but small wins can reignite your drive and keep you moving forward. These incremental achievements act as reminders of your progress and reinforce the behaviors needed to reach larger goals.

To create small wins, break your objectives into manageable steps. For instance, instead of focusing solely on losing a significant amount of weight, set weekly goals like drinking more water, increasing daily steps, or completing a set number of workouts. Each success, no matter how minor, builds confidence and provides a sense of accomplishment.

Acknowledging these wins is equally important. Celebrate your progress by treating yourself to something meaningful—perhaps a new workout playlist, a fitness gadget, or even a relaxing evening off. These rewards don't have to be extravagant but should feel like a genuine recognition of your effort.

Tracking your progress visually can also help reinforce motivation. Use a journal, chart, or app to log achievements and see how far you've come. This visual representation serves as a powerful reminder of your dedication and can inspire you during moments of doubt.

Finally, share your wins with others. Whether it's with a workout buddy, online community, or coach, celebrating together can amplify the joy and deepen your commitment to future goals.

## 3.3 Adapting to Life Changes and Challenges: Staying Consistent Amidst Unpredictability

Life is unpredictable, and adapting to changes is critical for maintaining your fitness journey. Whether it's a new job, family responsibilities, or unexpected events, having strategies to stay on track ensures that you can navigate challenges without abandoning your goals.

Start by reassessing your routines when circumstances shift. For example, if a new schedule limits your workout time, consider shorter, more efficient workouts or switching to home-based routines. Flexibility is key—adjusting your approach to fit your current situation allows you to maintain consistency even during busy or stressful periods.

Prioritize the habits that provide the most impact. When time or energy is limited, focus on essential behaviors like meal prep, hydration, or a quick daily walk. These foundational habits keep you connected to your goals, even if other aspects of your routine need to be temporarily scaled back.

Anticipate that challenges will arise and prepare contingency plans. For example, keep healthy snacks on hand for hectic days or create a list of quick workouts for when time is tight. Planning ahead reduces the likelihood of falling completely off track.

Most importantly, maintain a long-term perspective. Temporary disruptions are just that—temporary. By staying committed to your overall vision and adapting to life's ebbs and flows, you build resilience and ensure that progress continues, even in the face of adversity.

Overcoming setbacks, celebrating small wins, and adapting to life's challenges are integral to maintaining motivation and achieving lasting success. By focusing on these strategies, you'll navigate the ups and downs of your fitness journey with confidence and determination.

# Final Thoughts and Long-Term Success

## Reflecting on Your Journey

### 1.1 Reviewing Your Progress: Taking Stock of Your Achievements

As you approach the conclusion of your macro nutrition journey outlined in this book, it's important to pause and reflect on the progress you've made. Reflection is not just about measuring how far you've come but also about acknowledging the effort, commitment, and resilience it took to get here.

Start by revisiting your initial goals. Whether you aimed to lose weight, gain muscle, improve performance, or simply adopt healthier habits, take a moment to assess your achievements. Consider the tangible changes—perhaps you've reached a target weight, lifted heavier weights, or maintained consistent macro tracking for months. These milestones are proof of your hard work and dedication.

Equally important are the less visible accomplishments, like improved energy levels, a better relationship with food, or increased confidence in your ability to navigate challenges. These victories often have a profound impact on your overall well-being and are worth celebrating just as much as the physical results.

Reflection also allows you to identify areas for growth. Recognizing where you struggled—whether it was consistency, planning, or staying motivated—provides valuable insights for the future. Use this awareness to refine your strategies and set new, attainable goals moving forward.

Finally, celebrate your journey, no matter how imperfect it may have been. Progress is rarely linear, and every step forward, including overcoming setbacks, contributes to your success. Acknowledging your efforts fosters a positive mindset and motivates you to keep striving for your best self.

## 1.2 What You've Learned: Key Takeaways from This Journey

Throughout this book, you've gained knowledge and tools to take control of your nutrition and build lasting habits. Reflecting on what you've learned reinforces these concepts and ensures they become second nature in your daily life.

Consider the principles of macro tracking you've mastered, from understanding your unique nutritional needs to fine-tuning your intake for optimal results. Recall how you've learned to adapt to challenges, celebrate small wins, and maintain accountability. These skills are not just temporary strategies but life-changing practices that can be applied in many areas of health and fitness.

Beyond practical knowledge, think about the mindset shifts you've experienced. Perhaps you've developed greater patience, resilience, and self-compassion, realizing that progress takes time and setbacks are opportunities for growth. These mental shifts are just as crucial as the physical changes and serve as a foundation for long-term success.

Finally, recognize how far you've come in building a more informed and intentional approach to nutrition. By integrating the lessons from this book into your lifestyle, you've equipped yourself to continue thriving long after reaching your initial goals.

## 1.3 The Bigger Picture: Embracing Macro Nutrition as a Lifelong Journey

Macro nutrition isn't a short-term fix or a one-time experiment—it's a framework for sustaining health and achieving your best self over the course of your life. By viewing it as a lifelong journey rather than a destination, you open the door to continuous growth and adaptation.

Life is full of changes, from evolving priorities to unexpected challenges, and your approach to nutrition should adapt accordingly. The knowledge you've gained enables you to navigate these shifts with confidence, ensuring that your health remains a priority no matter the circumstances.

Moreover, the principles of macro tracking can be applied beyond personal fitness. Whether you're helping family members adopt healthier habits, sharing your journey with a supportive community, or simply leading by example, your commitment to macro nutrition has a ripple effect that inspires others.

The ultimate goal is not perfection but sustainability. By focusing on balance, flexibility, and consistency, you can maintain a healthy relationship with food and your body for years to come. Embrace the idea that this journey is ongoing and that every choice you make contributes to your well-being.

As you move forward, carry the lessons and successes of this book with you. Continue to reflect on your progress, adapt to life's changes, and celebrate the wins—both big and small. Macro nutrition isn't just about reaching a goal; it's about building a lifestyle that supports your health, happiness, and long-term success.

# Keeping Momentum Going

## 2.1 Maintaining Long-Term Results: Strategies for Consistency Over Time

Reaching your goals is a significant accomplishment, but maintaining those results is where true success lies. Sustaining long-term outcomes requires consistency, adaptability, and a commitment to the habits that got you here in the first place.

One key strategy is to establish routines that fit seamlessly into your life. By now, you've likely developed systems for meal prep, macro tracking, and regular exercise. Ensure these practices remain manageable and enjoyable by periodically assessing and tweaking them to fit your current lifestyle. For example, if a new job limits your time, adjust your meal prep to include simpler recipes or schedule shorter but effective workouts.

Consistency also hinges on having realistic expectations. Understand that maintaining results doesn't mean adhering to perfection every day. Life will inevitably include holidays, social events, and periods of lower motivation. Instead of striving for flawless adherence, focus on making mindful choices most of the time. This flexibility reduces stress and prevents burnout, making it easier to stay on track.

Another essential element is monitoring progress even after reaching your goals. Regular check-ins with your weight, body composition, or performance metrics can help you identify and address any shifts early on. Staying aware of your progress keeps you accountable and ensures you maintain the momentum you've built.

Finally, prioritize self-care and mental health. Long-term success isn't just about physical results; it's about feeling balanced, energized, and fulfilled. By keeping both physical and mental well-being at the forefront, you set yourself up for lasting success.

## 2.2 Embracing New Goals: Setting the Stage for Continued Growth

Once you've achieved your initial objectives, it's time to embrace new goals that keep you excited and motivated. Progress is an ongoing journey, and setting fresh challenges ensures you continue growing and evolving.

Start by reflecting on what excites you. Perhaps you want to focus on a new fitness pursuit, like running a marathon, improving strength, or mastering a sport. Alternatively, you might set goals beyond fitness, such as enhancing mental clarity, improving sleep quality, or learning new culinary skills to expand your healthy meal repertoire.

When setting new goals, make them specific, measurable, and time-bound. For instance, instead of vaguely aiming to "get stronger," target a specific lift or performance metric, such as squatting your body weight within three months. Clear objectives provide direction and a sense of purpose.

It's also crucial to balance challenge with realism. While ambitious goals are motivating, setting unrealistic expectations can lead to frustration. Choose objectives that push you outside your comfort zone but remain attainable with effort and consistency.

Finally, share your goals with others. Whether it's a coach, a fitness group, or a friend, having someone to support and celebrate your progress enhances your accountability and enjoyment of the journey.

## 2.3 Lifelong Nutrition: Shifting from Temporary Diets to Sustainable Lifestyles

The ultimate goal of this journey is to transition from seeing nutrition as a short-term project to embracing it as a lifelong lifestyle. Macro tracking isn't just about achieving a specific result; it's a tool for empowering you to make informed decisions and maintain balance in your daily life.

Adopting lifelong nutrition means prioritizing flexibility and sustainability. While there may be periods when you track macros diligently, there will also be times when you rely on intuition and the foundational knowledge you've built. Trust that you've internalized the principles of balance, portion control, and nutrient quality to guide your choices even without meticulous tracking.

One way to ensure this shift is to focus on building habits that align with your values and preferences. For example, if you enjoy experimenting with recipes, continue exploring healthy yet satisfying meals. If you thrive on structure, maintain a loose framework for meal planning that keeps you organized without feeling restrictive.

It's also essential to view nutrition within the broader context of your life. Your dietary habits should support not only physical health but also social, emotional, and mental well-being. This might mean occasionally indulging in treats without guilt or adapting your approach to accommodate different life stages and goals.

By committing to lifelong nutrition, you embrace a mindset of balance, flexibility, and growth. Instead of chasing fleeting diets or short-term results, you cultivate a sustainable way of living that supports your health, happiness, and overall quality of life.

As you move forward, remember that maintaining momentum, setting new goals, and adopting a lifestyle approach to nutrition are the cornerstones of long-term success. With these strategies in place, you're well-equipped to continue thriving and enjoying the journey ahead.

# The Path Forward

## 3.1 Continuing to Evolve: Embracing Change in Your Nutrition and Goals

The journey toward health and fitness doesn't end with achieving a single goal—it's a continuous process of evolution. As your life changes, so will your nutritional needs, fitness goals, and priorities. Recognizing and embracing this natural progression is key to sustaining long-term success.

Over time, your focus may shift from weight loss to muscle building, or from performance-based goals to overall wellness. For instance, younger athletes might prioritize optimizing performance, while older individuals might emphasize maintaining bone density or managing chronic conditions. These shifts are a normal part of life, and adapting your approach ensures your habits stay aligned with your needs.

Regularly reevaluating your goals helps you stay on track. Set aside time every few months to assess your current priorities and determine if your strategies need adjustment. For example, if you notice that your energy levels have dipped or your workouts feel stagnant, it might be time to revisit your macro ratios or try a new fitness program.

It's also important to stay curious and open to learning. Nutrition science continues to evolve, and new research or techniques may refine your understanding of what works best for you. Keeping an adaptable mindset ensures that your approach remains effective and engaging as your circumstances change.

## 3.2 Seeking Help When Needed: The Value of Professional Support

While self-guided progress is empowering, there may be times when seeking help from professionals can accelerate your success or provide clarity during challenging moments. Recognizing when to ask for support is not a sign of weakness but rather a proactive step toward achieving your goals.

Registered dietitians, nutrition coaches, and fitness trainers offer valuable expertise tailored to your unique needs. If you're struggling to adjust your macros, experiencing plateaus, or facing health issues, these professionals can provide personalized guidance and evidence-based strategies.

Support isn't limited to professionals. Leaning on community resources, such as fitness groups, online forums, or friends with similar goals, can provide encouragement and accountability. Sharing your experiences and learning from others fosters a sense of connection and shared purpose.

Additionally, mental health professionals can be instrumental if emotional eating, stress, or other psychological factors impact your nutrition. Addressing these challenges holistically ensures that your journey is sustainable and fulfilling.

Seeking help is a sign of commitment to your well-being. It shows that you're willing to invest in your success and use all available resources to achieve your best self.

## 3.3 Staying Empowered: Owning Your Nutrition and Progress

Ultimately, the most important takeaway from this journey is recognizing that you hold the power to shape your nutrition and progress. Every choice you make, whether big or small, contributes to your overall health and success.

This sense of empowerment is the foundation for long-term achievement.

One way to stay empowered is by trusting your ability to make informed decisions. Over the course of this book, you've gained the knowledge and tools to navigate the complexities of macro nutrition with confidence. Whether you're meal planning, dining out, or adjusting your intake, you now have the skills to adapt and thrive in any situation.

Celebrate your autonomy by embracing the flexibility and balance that macro tracking offers. Remember that you're not tied to rigid rules; instead, you have the freedom to make choices that align with your goals and lifestyle. This perspective transforms nutrition from a chore into a meaningful, enjoyable practice.

Finally, remind yourself of your resilience. There will be challenges, but each obstacle is an opportunity to grow stronger and more determined. Trust in your ability to overcome setbacks and adapt to life's changes.

Staying empowered means taking ownership of your journey and recognizing that you're in control of your health, happiness, and future. With this mindset, you'll not only achieve lasting success but also inspire others to take charge of their own paths forward.

As you continue evolving, seeking help when needed, and embracing your empowerment, you solidify the foundation for a lifetime of progress and fulfillment. The path forward is yours to create—step into it with confidence and purpose.

# Summary

As you reach the end of this journey, remember that the blueprint for success isn't just about knowledge—it's about action. The principles of macronutrient balance, strategic adjustments, and sustainable habits outlined in Macro Hacks For Men are your tools for creating lasting change.

Your fitness goals, whether they involve losing fat, building muscle, or maintaining a healthy lifestyle, are deeply personal. They require patience, persistence, and a commitment to learning what works best for your unique needs. By embracing macronutrient-focused nutrition, you empower yourself to fuel your body purposefully and align your efforts with your objectives.

Start by defining clear, measurable goals. Use the methods shared in this book to calculate your Total Daily Energy Expenditure (TDEE) and tailor your macro ratios accordingly. Track your intake, listen to your body, and refine your approach through trial and error. Consistency, not perfection, is the foundation of progress.

Meal planning and preparation are your allies in a busy world. From grocery lists to batch cooking, these small yet impactful practices ensure you're always equipped with the right fuel. Balance is key—allow flexibility for celebrations and life's inevitable surprises without losing sight of your long-term vision.

Above all, this is a lifestyle, not a temporary fix. Fitness is a marathon, not a sprint. As your body and goals evolve, so will your needs. Periodically reassess your progress, adjust your macros, and continue educating yourself about nutrition and health. With each adjustment, you're honing a system that works for you—one that delivers not only physical results but also mental clarity and confidence.

Macro Hacks For Men is more than a guide; it's an invitation to take control of your health and unlock your potential. The journey doesn't end here—it begins now. Go forward with purpose, armed with the knowledge to build your best body, and remember that every choice you make brings you closer to the best version of yourself.